D0836794

Mosby's
Biomedical Science Series

UNDERSTANDING
Immunology

Mosby's
Biomedical Science Series

UNDERSTANDING
Immunology

NANCY COE CLOUGH, DVM, PhD

Veterinary Medical Officer

Center for Veterinary Biologics

USDA-APHIS

Ames, Iowa

JAMES A. ROTH, DVM, PhD

Professor of Immunology

College of Veterinary Medicine

Iowa State University

Ames, Iowa

With 40 Illustrations

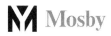 Mosby

St. Louis Baltimore Boston Carlsbad Chicago Naples New York Philadelphia Portland
London Madrid Mexico City Singapore Sydney Tokyo Toronto Wiesbaden

AHE 1188

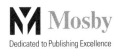 Mosby

Dedicated to Publishing Excellence

A Times Mirror
Company

Publisher: Don E. Ladig
Executive Editor: Paul W. Pratt
Senior Developmental Editor: Teri Merchant
Project Manager: Mark Spann
Production Editor: Anne Salmo
Book Design Manager: Judi Lang
Manufacturing Manager: Betty Mueller
Cover Designer: Teresa Breckwoldt

Copyright © 1998 by Mosby-Year Book, Inc.

All rights reserved. No part of this publication may be reproduced,
stored in a retrieval system, or transmitted, in any form or by any
means, electronic, mechanical, photocopying, recording, or otherwise,
without written permission from the publisher.

Permission to photocopy or reproduce solely for internal or personal
use is permitted for libraries or other users registered with the Copyright
Clearance Center, provided that the base fee of $4.00 per chapter plus $.10
per page is paid directly to the Copyright Clearance Center, 222 Rosewood
Drive, Danvers, MA 01923. This consent does not extend to other kinds
of copying, such as copying for general distribution, for advertising or
promotional purposes, for creating new collected works, or for resale.

Printed in the United States of America
Composition by Carlisle Communications, Ltd.
Printing/binding by R.R. Donnelley & Sons Company

Mosby-Year Book, Inc.
11830 Westline Industrial Drive
St. Louis, Missouri 63146

Library of Congress Cataloging in Publication Data
Coe Clough, Nancy.
    Understanding immunology / Nancy Coe Clough, James A. Roth.
        p.   cm. —(Mosby's biomedical science series)
    Includes bibliographical references and index.
    ISBN 0-8151-8582-0
    1. Immunology.   2. Immunity.   3. Immune response.   I. Roth, James
A.   II. Title.   III. Series.
    [DNLM: 1. Immune System.   2. Immunity.   QW 504 C672u 1997]
    QR181.C713   1997 *1998*
    616.07'9—dc21
    DNLM/DLC
    for Library of Congress   97-9892
                                                                CIP

98 99 00 01 02/ 9 8 7 6 5 4 3 2 1

LSON LIBRARY
NORTHERN MICHIGAN UNIVERSITY
MARQUETTE MICHIGAN 49855

Preface

The authors' goal in writing this monograph was to give the reader an understanding of the basic principles underlying the ability of the immune system to protect an individual from disease and the mechanisms by which the immune system sometimes contributes to disease processes. The target audience for this monograph is students who are being exposed to immunology for the first time or medical professionals who want a quick update of the fundamental principles of immunology. The authors consider this book a PRE-text. It is intended to introduce the subject of immunology and convey an understanding of basic principles so that readers can more readily comprehend and integrate the material when they read a more conventional and detailed immunology text.

Immunology is a complex subject. It is difficult to know where to begin the study of immunology because all of the components of the immune system interact extensively. It is difficult to explain one component of the immune system without referring to the other components as though the student already was familiar with and understood them.

This text should give readers a quick overview and convey an understanding of the major principles of immunology without becoming mired in extensive detail. Detail is very important to the thorough understanding of immunology; however, it must come later in the learning process. Many excellent texts are available that thoroughly cover the field of immunology.

Immunology is a rapidly changing field. Discoveries continue to be made and occasionally improve the fundamental understanding of basic immunological concepts. We hope that this introductory text will convey an understanding of the principles of immunology and will stimulate readers' interest and prepare them for further study of the fascinating field of immunology.

Nancy Coe Clough

James A. Roth

Series Preface

Science textbooks are commonly entitled "Principles of . . ." Yet almost all of these books go far beyond principles to specify so much detail that they often obscure the principles. Too often the emphasis is on currently accepted facts, with principles used only to illustrate the facts, rather than using the minimum amount of fact to illustrate principles.

This situation argues for a new kind of textbook, one that focuses on the first principles of the discipline. In addition to encyclopedic tomes for each discipline, we need small texts that give the big picture and explicitly describe the basic foundational principles of the discipline—and no more!

As a start to what I hope will be a new movement in science education we are initiating a series of biomedical science teaching books that really are about principles. These books aim to be quick, yet elegant, overviews of the essence of the respective disciplines. The newcomer to the subject should find the preparation needed to understand the more comprehensive and detailed traditional textbooks and research journals. Maybe even highly specialized experts can find some useful perspectives from this approach. Senior people tend to get wrapped up in the details of their specialty and sometimes take the principles for granted.

We must have some kind of working definition of "principle." While many ways can express the idea, this Series of texts uses the following working definition:

> A principle must go beyond a collection of observations. Principles integrate multiple observations and help to explain these observations, providing understanding and insight. A principle embodies the underlying rules or mechanisms of structure, organization, or operation that give rise to the observations. We distinguish principles from concepts only in the sense that concepts often embody more than one principle.

In identifying these principles, we must recognize that they are basic tenets; i.e., commonly held *beliefs* about what is true and fundamental. Not everyone will agree that each of these "principles" deserves such lofty status. However, there is a fine line between principle and theory. Theories serve to inspire better theories that can establish principles more firmly.

Many of the statements of principle are incomplete. They may also lack sufficient qualification. Statements of principles serve to inspire more complete or precise exposition. The effort to identify principles comes at a cost: arbitrariness, uncertainty, controversy—but the cost is worth the price. *The search for principles is the Holy Grail of science.*

The practical value of such texts may lie in their pedagogical approach, which is the opposite from the tack taken in many textbooks on biological and medical subjects. Students are fed up with encyclopedic subjects. Students and professors alike are tired of an educational process devoted to pouring information into one ear while it spills out the other. The exponential expansion of new knowledge is causing cognitive overload in students and professors, short-circuiting their ability to sustain perspective about the whole of biomedical science and to think coherently about the details of how the body works in both health and disease. We are learning more and more about less and less, and that causes a progressive loss of capacity for synthesis and ability to think about the larger meanings of biomedical science. The texts in this series require the student to be actively involved in completing missing detail and providing the qualifications of special relevance.

Why These Books Are Needed

- Traditional texts are too big, too detailed, too indigestible
- Biomedical information is accumulating faster than students can handle
- Students are learning more and more about less and less
- Students, and even teachers, have trouble discerning the "must know" from the "nice to know"
- The new emphasis in teaching of biomedical sciences will be on how to manage, integrate, and apply information. That requires identification and understanding of the basic principles of the discipline

The advantages of books in this Series, as I see it, are as follows:

Advantages to Students:

- Students more likely to "see the forest instead of the trees"
  - What is important is made explicit
  - Cognitive overload can't obscure perspective and insight

- "Less is More"
  - Less material is easier to comprehend and remember
  - It is easier to remember unifying principles and concepts
  - Understanding principles empowers students to get more from new information
- Promotes active learning, critical thinking, insight, understanding
- Very useful in self-paced or collaborative learning paradigms
  - Helps assure that students have the required background
  - Students are better prepared to understand what they read in journals and reference books—with minimal help from professors
- Books are smaller, cost less, are more portable, and are easier to peruse
- High portability and condensed nature encourage frequent review
- Longer half-life
  - Traditional texts are out of date as soon as printed
  - Principles are "eternal"

Benefits to Professors

- Allows specialized instruction with less fear that basics are being missed
- After mastering principles, students are equally prepared for subsequent instruction
- Enlivens the lecture period. Meaningful discussion and debate facilitated

Benefits to Graduates

- Quick way to review latest concepts, especially in fields in which they have not kept up
- "User-friendly" access to specialties or to especially complex disciplines

As professors increasingly recognize, the proliferation of research literature has made it difficult to decide what is fundamental about their discipline that must be taught to students. The books in this Series aim to help professors identify that core understanding. Even where a professor may disagree with certain statements of principle, the books provide a focus and a stimulus to the professor to refine those statements of principle with which they disagree.

Where professors believe that more factual detail is needed, they can provide it or direct students to it with some reassurance that students still understand the central core of the discipline. Thus, these books can substitute for the standard, fact-filled§ textbook and give professors the flexibility to use other instructional media, such as computer-assisted instruction, journal articles, and even standard textbooks as reference sources to complement Mosby's Biomedical Science Series.

Books in this Series would seem especially important for curricula that stress problem- or case-based learning (PBL). In recognition of the cognitive overload problem some medical schools (McMasters, Harvard, Southern Illinois, Bowman Gray, University of New Mexico) have pioneered in converting the traditional lecture-based curriculum to a tutorial, group-based learning format where critical thinking and information management skills are emphasized rather than rote memory. Some veterinary colleges are also making similar curricular changes. This trend will surely grow, because it is aimed at teaching students to *manage* and *integrate* an ever-expanding biomedical data base.

However, many institutions have thoughtfully considered but rejected PBL-type curricula out of fear that students will have huge gaps in their understanding of core biomedical science disciplines. Books in this Series not only help PBL students to know what the fundamental principles are but also present those principles in a quick and easily digestible form. Understanding these principles increases the likelihood that PBL students will truly understand what they read in journals and reference books as they try to apply it to clinical cases or academic problems.

Organization of These Books

The first—and most difficult—part of writing this kind of text is the identification and terse statement of the first principles of a discipline. Then the principles are consolidated, if necessary, and grouped into categories to make it easier to organize and remember them.

Each category has an Introduction that states the principles in that category. The authors treat each principle as a topic that states the principle and identifies its category. Then the principle is explained, including the use of one or more examples, accompanied by one or two diagrams or pictures. Another section defines key terms, and yet another lists other principles that are most directly related. Finally, a reference section lists several key references. At the end of the topics in a given category, a review section presents some study questions.

W. R. (Bill) Klemm
Series Editor
Texas A & M University
College Station, Texas

Contents

Introduction to the Immune System

The immune system is responsible for protecting individuals from infectious diseases, parasites, cancer, and the effects of certain toxins. It has many potent cellular and molecular mechanisms for carrying out its protective function. Under certain conditions the immune system may react inappropriately, resulting in significant damage to normal tissue (a hypersensitivity disease).

This first chapter will give an overview of the major characteristics of the immune system and some of the ways in which the components of the immune system are categorized.

TOPIC 1: Overview of Immunology

Principles

1. Immunity to disease is due to a complex set of physical barriers to infection, the actions of white blood cells (leukocytes), and the presence of a variety of protective molecules in body fluids and on body surfaces.
2. Some of the components of immunity are naturally present in individuals (natural immunity). Others are only present if the individual has been previously exposed to the particular infectious agent (acquired immunity).
3. An infectious agent or any molecule that induces an acquired immune response is called an antigen.
4. The acquired immune response takes several days to develop after the first exposure to antigen and is due to antibodies produced through the actions of B lymphocytes (humoral immunity) and/or to cell-mediated immunity produced through the actions of

T lymphocytes. The immune response occurs more rapidly when the individual is exposed to the same antigen a second time. This is called immunological memory.

5. Acquired immunity may be passively acquired through the transfer of antibodies or T lymphocytes from one individual to another, or it may be actively produced (acquired) by the individual's own lymphoid system.

6. The immune system can exhibit tolerance. The immune system distinguishes an individual's own antigens from foreign antigens so that the immune system does not normally attack molecules and cells that are normal components of healthy tissues.

7. If the immune system is slow or deficient in its activity, the individual is more susceptible to infectious diseases and/or cancer. Conversely, if the immune system overreacts to antigens, or reacts to normal self antigens, it can cause damage and hypersensitivity disease.

Explanation

The immune system protects individuals from infectious diseases, the effects of certain toxins, and cancer (neoplastic diseases). To do this, the immune system must be able to rapidly distinguish between cells and molecules that normally belong in the body (referred to as "self") and cells and molecules that do not normally belong in the body (referred to as "non-self"). Resistance to infectious diseases, toxins, and cancer is brought about by various physical and chemical barriers to infection, the actions of white blood cells, and the actions of a variety of molecules in body fluids and on cell surfaces. The term immunity comes from the Latin word *immunis,* meaning free or exempt. An individual who is immune is free or exempt from the effects of pathogenic organisms or toxins. *Immunology* is the study of the immune system, which is composed of a wide variety of cellular and molecular components working in concert to bring about resistance to disease.

The state of being immune may be absolute. For example, members of one species are often not susceptible to viruses that cause disease in a different species. For those diseases to which a species is susceptible, the level of immunity is usually not absolute. The individual may not be truly immune but rather may be relatively resistant to the disease. The individual with immune resistance may get a mild form of disease instead of a severe form of disease. A high dose of infectious agents or sufficient stresses on the immune system may overwhelm the ability of the immune system to resist infection, and the individual may develop a disease despite the level of immunity that has developed.

There are several useful ways of classifying immunity. These include natural immunity vs. acquired immunity, passive immunity vs. active immunity, and humoral immunity vs. cell-mediated immunity.

Natural immunity and acquired immunity

Natural immunity is due to a variety of mechanisms that do not depend on previous exposure to infectious agents. Infectious agents and other substances to which the immune system responds are referred to as *antigens*. The natural immune mechanisms are present and may provide resistance to disease immediately on first exposure to infectious agents. The mechanisms that are responsible for natural immunity include phago-cytic white blood cells, complement proteins, antimicrobial compounds in body fluids, and physical barriers to infection, such as the skin and mucous membranes (see the box on this page). People and animals have some degree of natural immunity to nearly all infectious agents. This natural resistance can be overwhelmed if the natural defense mechanisms are impaired or if the individual is exposed to a high concentration of infectious agents.

■■■ Native and Acquired ■■■
Immune Defense Mechanisms

The native defense mechanisms do not require previous exposure to antigen to be effective and can function rapidly on first exposure to antigen. The acquired immune defense mechanisms are highly antigen specific and require 1 to 2 weeks after first exposure to antigen to be fully active.

Native Defense Mechanisms:

Physical barriers and impediments to infection:
- Intact skin and mucous membranes
- Normal microbial flora
- Fatty acids in the skin
- Acid in the stomach
- Mucociliary escalator in the trachea
- Enzymes in intestine, saliva, tears
- Coughing, sneezing, vomiting, diarrhea
- Fever

Antimicrobial components of native defense:
- Complement system
- Type I interferon
- Phagocytic cells

Continued

■ Native and Acquired ■
Immune Defense Mechanisms — cont'd

- Acute phase proteins
- Cationic peptides on epithelial surfaces
- Natural killer lymphocytes

Acquired Immune Defense Mechanisms:

Antibodies produced by B lymphocytes:

- IgM
- IgG
- IgA
- IgE

Cell-mediated immunity:

- Cytokines produced by T lymphocytes
- Cytotoxic T lymphocytes

Acquired immunity requires previous exposure to an infectious agent or to a vaccine containing antigens from the infectious agent. Acquired immunity is a result of B and/or T lymphocyte responses to the antigen and takes several days to develop after the first exposure to the antigen (primary immune response). B and T lymphocytes will respond much more rapidly the second time that the same antigen is encountered (secondary immune response). This is called *immunological memory*. Acquired immunity is due to antibodies produced through the actions of B lymphocytes or cell-mediated immunity produced through the actions of T lymphocytes. An individual with acquired immunity to a particular disease has a greater degree of resistance than an individual who has only natural immunity.

Passive immunity and active immunity

Passive immunity is a special type of acquired immunity in which the individual passively receives either antibodies or lymphocytes from another individual who has already developed an immune response to an antigen. The most common example of passive immunity is the passage of antibody from the mother to the offspring through the placenta or milk. Without this passive transfer of immunity, the newborn would have only natural immunity and no acquired immune mechanisms to help it to resist the diseases to which it may be exposed very soon after birth. Passive immunity wanes after a few weeks or months and must be replaced with an individual's own active immune response, which can be much longer lasting, to keep the individual healthy.

Active immunity is a form of acquired immunity in which the individual's own B or T lymphocytes respond to the presence of antigens and produce an antibody and/or cell-mediated immune response. Several days are required after first exposure to an antigen before active immunity is fully developed.

Humoral immunity and cell-mediated immunity

Early in the study of immunity it was observed that resistance to some diseases could be passively transferred from an immune animal to a nonimmune animal by transferring serum. This was called *humoral immunity* because it was due to the transference of the liquid portion of blood, not the cellular portion (*humores* is a Latin term for "a liquid"). We now know that the passive transfer of humoral immunity was due to the presence of specific antibodies in the serum.

Immunity to some other types of diseases could only be transferred from an immune animal to a nonimmune animal by transferring the cellular portion of blood. This type of immunity was called *cell-mediated immunity*. It is now known that this was due to the transfer of T lymphocytes. It is now also appreciated that antibodies and T lymphocytes are both important for resistance to most diseases and that their production and activity are linked. However, the classifications of humoral and cell-mediated immunity are still useful for understanding disease resistance.

The immune system can be very aggressive and powerful in eliminating cells and molecules that are identified as foreign. To do this, the immune system must distinguish between the myriad cells and molecules that are "self" and are normally present in an individual from cells and molecules that are not normally present. The ability to distinguish between "self" and "non-self" arises primarily during development of the immune system in the fetus. Lymphocytes that arise during development in the fetus that would recognize and attack "self" antigens are eliminated or suppressed. Consequently, the mature immune system does not normally attack molecules and cells that are normal components of healthy tissues. Lymphocytes that are capable of detecting antigens that are not present in the fetus proceed to mature and circulate in the individual after birth so that they can detect and respond to foreign antigens that may invade. Occasionally, in some individuals the ability of the immune system to distinguish self from non-self becomes impaired, and the immune system may attack normal cells or molecules present in the body. This produces damage to tissues and organs and can result in disease referred to as *autoimmune disease*. Even when the immune system responds to foreign antigens, it can cause damage to host cells and tissues associated with the foreign antigens. When symptoms of disease are due to the actions of the immune system, the diseases are referred to as *hypersensitivity diseases.*

Immunology is a very rapidly evolving field. The cellular and molecular mechanisms responsible for immunity are rapidly being elucidated. These basic science advances in the understanding of the immune system hold tremendous promise for disease prevention and therapy.

Related Topics

Recognition of self vs. non-self
Memory lymphocytes
Autoimmunity
Hypersensitivities

Additional Reading

Male, D. and Roitt, I. 1996. Chapter 1. Introduction to the immune system. In Roitt, I., Brostoff, J., and Male, D. (eds.) Immunology, 4th ed. Mosby-Year Book, St. Louis.

Rich, R.R. 1996. Chapter 1. The human immune response. In Rich, R.R. (ed.) Clinical Immunology: Principles and Practice. Mosby-Year Book, St. Louis.

TERMS

Antibody	Protein molecules produced by B cells and plasma cells in response to specific antigens to which they will bind. Antibodies are also called immunoglobulins.
Antigen	Molecules or cells that induce the production of antibodies and/or a T cell-mediated immune response by binding to specific receptors on lymphocyte surfaces.
Autoimmune Disease	Disease that is due to the immune response targeting "self" tissues.
B Lymphocytes	White blood cells that are produced and mature in the bone marrow of mammals, circulate between the blood and lymphoid tissues, and are responsible for production of antibodies.
Cell-mediated Immunity	Immunity brought about by the action of T lymphocytes secreting cytokines or acting as cytotoxic cells.

Complement	A group of proteins in the plasma that forms an enzyme cascade that may be activated rapidly by invading pathogens. Complement activation initiates an inflammatory response and a series of events that help to control many infectious agents.
Hypersensitivity Diseases	Diseases in which the major clinical symptoms are due to the immune response to an antigen.
Immunological Memory	The phenomenon by which the immune response is more rapid and aggressive the second and subsequent times that an individual is exposed to an antigen. Also called the anamnestic response.
Immunological Tolerance	The phenomenon by which the immune system specifically does not respond to certain antigens, especially normal "self" antigens.
Phagocytosis	The process by which particulate material, such as a bacterium, is ingested by a cell, which typically will then attempt to destroy the particle.
T Lymphocytes	White blood cells that are produced in the bone marrow, mature under the influence of the thymus gland, circulate between the blood and lymphoid tissues, and are responsible for producing cell-mediated immunity.

Study Questions

1. What are some natural protective mechanisms in the respiratory tract? The gastrointestinal tract?
2. Would you expect an individual to be protected from a disease immediately after receiving his or her first dose of vaccine? Why?
3. What would happen if immunological tolerance to self antigens broke down?
4. What is immunological memory?
5. Compare and contrast natural and acquired immunity.

CHAPTER 2

Components of the Immune System

Many different cell types and molecules contribute to host defense and are considered part of the immune system. Each of these components of the immune system has unique aspects in the way they are triggered, their biological effects, and in the mechanisms they use to control invading pathogens or aberrant cells (cancer cells). All of these components have certain aspects of their function that can be activated rapidly on first exposure to an invading pathogen to help control it. These rapid responses are important for controlling an infection while the B and T lymphocytes are beginning to respond to produce acquired immunity. The immediate defense components of the complement system, the phagocytic system, and the lymphoid system (the natural killer lymphocytes) all work much more efficiently in the presence of humoral immunity (antibodies) and cell-mediated immunity (cytokines), which require 1 to 2 weeks to develop after initial exposure.

In this chapter we present core concepts about each of the major components of the immune system. These components are the white blood cells, the complement system, the phagocytic cells, and the lymphoid system. Extensive interaction among these various components of the immune system is a hallmark of immune system activity.

List of Principles

The White Blood Cells Five basic types of white blood cells (leukocytes) work together to resist invasion by pathogens and to control
Continued

List of Principles — cont'd

cancer cells that may arise. All of the white blood cells are produced predominately in the bone marrow, circulate through the blood, and may eventually be found in the tissues.

B and T lymphocytes are the only cells in the body capable of highly specific recognition of antigen.

Neutrophils, monocytes (macrophages), eosinophils, basophils (mast cells), and natural killer lymphocytes are part of the native defense mechanisms and can help to fight infection rapidly after the first exposure to an infectious agent. Their activity is enhanced by the presence of specific antibody or memory T cells that recognize the antigen.

The Complement System

The complement system is an enzyme cascade system present in the plasma that can respond rapidly to attack some infectious agents and focus defense mechanisms at the site of infection. The complement cascade can be triggered by some microbial surfaces and by some antigen-antibody complexes.

Because the complement system involves an enzyme cascade, a small initiating signal can trigger a rapid and aggressive response. This is called *biological amplification.*

Activation of the complement system may help to control bacterial infection by damaging the bacterial membrane, attracting neutrophils to the site of infection, increasing blood flow to the site of infection (vasodilation), facilitating leakage of plasma proteins into the site of infection (increased vascular permeability), and opsonizing bacteria for phagocytosis.

Excessive activation of the complement system can lead to tissue damage.

Phagocytic Cells

A major immunological defense mechanism is phagocytosis, which is the process whereby particles are internalized into certain cells.

A bacterial infection generates chemical factors that attract large numbers of neutrophils to the site of infection in a few hours and that cause the bone marrow to rapidly release more neutrophils into the circulation.

Phagocytic cells are an important part of the native defense mechanisms for protecting against bacterial infection before the humoral and cell-mediated immune systems have time to react. However, phagocytic cells can be much more efficient

==
■■■■■■■■■■ **List of Principles — cont'd** ■■■■■■■
==

and effective with the help of antibody and T-cell cytokines.

Phagocytic cells kill bacteria that they have ingested (phago-cytized) using the contents of their lysosomes and toxic oxygen and nitrogen metabolites generated during phagocytosis.

Genetic defects in phagocytic cell function or decreased phagocytic cell function caused by stress, viral infection, or drug therapy leads to increased susceptibility to bacterial infection.

Neutrophils recruited to inflammatory sites may contribute to tissue damage.

Macrophages play a very important role as antigen-presenting cells to T lymphocytes.

The Lymphoid System

Lymphocytes that react with self antigens are eliminated dur-ing development in primary lymphoid tissues.

Organized secondary lymphoid tissues (e.g., lymph nodes and spleen) are sites where antigens are collected and presented to lymphocytes.

Lymphocytes circulate between blood and lymphoid tissues to optimize their chances for encountering antigens.

TOPIC 1: The White Blood Cells

Principles

1. Five basic types of white blood cells (leukocytes) work together to resist invasion by pathogens and to control cancer cells that may arise. All of the white blood cells are produced predominately in the bone marrow, circulate through the blood, and eventually may be found in the tissues.

2. B and T lymphocytes are the only cells in the body capable of highly specific recognition of antigen.

3. Neutrophils, monocytes (macrophages), eosinophils, basophils (mast cells), and natural killer lymphocytes are part of the native defense mechanisms and can help to fight infection rapidly during the first exposure to an infectious agent. Their activity is enhanced by the presence of specific antibody or memory T cells, which recognize the antigen.

Explanation

Five basic types of white blood cells (leukocytes) can be found circulating in the bloodstream: neutrophils, basophils, eosinophils, monocytes, and lymphocytes (Table 2-1). All five types are produced in the bone marrow from a common progenitor stem cell. This stem cell in the bone marrow continually replicates. The daughter cells gradually differentiate through several series of divisions to produce the five types of white blood cells, as well as the red blood cells and platelets. Mature white blood cells are released from the bone marrow into the bloodstream, where they circulate for varying lengths of time. Neutrophils, monocytes, eosinophils, and basophils eventually enter the tissues and do not return to the bloodstream. These cells are not specific for certain antigens. B and T lymphocytes are specific for certain antigens and circulate between the blood and the lymphoid tissues in search of those antigens that they recognize.

Neutrophils, eosinophils, and basophils have a lobulated nucleus and are called *polymorphonuclear leukocytes*. These cells also have granules in their cytoplasm and are sometimes called *granulocytes*. Neutrophil granules do not stain with the typical hematoxylin and eosin stain used on blood smears (neutral staining). Eosinophils have large granules that stain red with eosin dye. Basophils have large granules that have a basic pH and stain blue with hematoxylin dye. Lymphocytes and monocytes have a typical round or oval (sometimes indented) nucleus and are called *mononuclear leukocytes*. Monocytes are usually larger than lymphocytes.

Neutrophils are phagocytic cells that form the first line of defense primarily against bacterial infections, but they can also play a role in certain viral infections. They make up a high percentage of the circulating white blood cells and spend only a few hours in the bloodstream before migrating into the tissues. Therefore, to meet the demands of high turnover, they are produced in much larger numbers in the bone marrow than the other white blood cell types.

Neutrophils are attracted rapidly and in large numbers to sites of bacterial infection and significantly contribute to the inflammatory process. There is a large pool of mature neutrophils in the bone marrow that can be released into the bloodstream rapidly in response to inflammatory signals. If the inflammatory signals are strong, then immature neutrophils can also be released into the bloodstream. The immature cells have an unlobulated horseshoe-shaped nucleus and are called *band cells*. (The mature neutrophils are sometimes called "segs" because of their segmented nucleus). The presence of many band cells (and usually a high total neutrophil count) in the blood generally indicates that an acute inflammatory process is under way.

TABLE 2-1   DISTRIBUTION, HALF-LIFE IN THE CIRCULATION, AND MAJOR FUNCTIONS OF LEUKOCYTES IN HUMANS

Leukocyte	Approximate Percentage of Total Leukocytes	Approximate Half-Life in Circulation	Major Functions
Neutrophils	60%	8 hours	Phagocytosis and killing of bacteria
Eosinophils	2%-5%	13 hours	Attack migrating parasites, control products of mast cell degranulation
Basophils	<1%	≈ 1 week	Release histamine and vasoactive substances
Monocytes	10%	3 days	Become macrophages; phagocytosis and antigen presentation
Lymphocytes	25%	Recirculate between blood and lymphatics	Acquired immunity
Lymphocyte Subsets	**As an Approximate Percentage of Total Lymphocytes**		**Major Functions**
T helper	55%		Secrete cytokines
T cytotoxic	25%		Kill cells expressing foreign antigens
B	10%		Produce antibodies
NK	10%		Kill cells not expressing normal self antigens

Neutrophils have receptors for antibody molecules that have bound to antigens. This enables the neutrophils to specifically bind to and attack those antigens. Some cytokines produced by T lymphocytes and monocytes are able to activate the neutrophil to be more aggressive and efficient in killing infectious agents.

Basophils are present in the bloodstream in very low numbers, usually 1% to 2% of the total white blood cells or less. Basophils are believed to migrate into the tissues and become mast cells. Mast cells are found primarily in the subcutaneous and submucosal tissues, where they are sentinels to monitor for invasion by parasites. Mast cells react to the presence of parasites by secreting substances that initiate inflammation and attract eosinophils to attack the parasites. Mast cells detect the presence of parasites because of immunoglobulin E (IgE) class antibody, which becomes bound to the parasite surface. Mast cells have receptors in their membrane specific for IgE. Mast cells respond after binding antigens through IgE by rapidly releasing their granule contents to the exterior of the cell. These granules contain high concentrations of histamine, serotonin, and other vasoactive amines, which cause vasodilation and increased vascular permeability. These two effects result in increased blood flow to the area and leakage of plasma components, including antibody and complement, into the tissues, as well as facilitated travel of white blood cells across the endothelial barrier into the tissues. Mast cell degranulation also attracts eosinophils to the site, where they may attack a parasite directly and/or inactivate the products of mast cell degranulation and thereby limit inflammatory damage.

Eosinophils are found in the bloodstream in low numbers in normal people and animals (0% to 10% of total leukocytes). The number in the circulation will increase in individuals who are heavily parasitized or who have certain types of allergies (type 1 hypersensitivities). Eosinophils play an important role in controlling migrating parasites and reducing the effects of mast cell degranulation. Eosinophils can inactivate some of the inflammatory factors released by mast cells, thereby limiting the damage caused by mast cell degranulation in certain types of allergies. Eosinophils have receptors on their membrane for the IgE antibody molecule. This allows eosinophils to attach to IgE bound to parasites so that they can more efficiently make contact with, and kill, the parasite.

Monocytes make up approximately 2% to 5% of the leukocytes in the peripheral blood. They circulate in the blood for a day or two, then migrate into the tissues to become macrophages. They may become specialized macrophages in specific tissues, such as Kupffer cells in the liver, microglial cells in the brain, or alveolar macrophages in the lung, or they may be wandering macrophages, which are found in nearly all tissues. Macrophages are important for controlling facultative intracellular bacterial infections, some viral infections, and some fungal infections.

They also play a very important role in trapping and processing antigens for presentation to T lymphocytes. Macrophages may survive for several weeks or months in normal tissues. They accumulate in large numbers at sites of chronic inflammation. On responding to infection or other inflammatory stimuli, they secrete cytokines, which are important cofactors for B and T lymphocyte responses to antigens. Antibodies can enhance macrophage function by coating (opsonizing) infectious agents, which will improve their ingestion and killing by macrophages. Cytokines secreted by T lymphocytes can activate macrophages to make them much more aggressive and efficient at killing intracellular pathogens.

Lymphocytes in the bloodstream in mammals are of three types: B lymphocytes, T lymphocytes, and natural killer (NK) lymphocytes. B lymphocytes are responsible for producing antibody, T lymphocytes are responsible for cell-mediated immunity, and NK lymphocytes are components of native immunity whose activity can be enhanced by the presence of antibody and certain cytokines. B lymphocytes were so named because they were discovered to be dependent on the bursa of Fabricius in birds for maturation. T lymphocytes are dependent on the thymus gland for maturation. Natural killer lymphocytes were so named because they are active naturally without previous exposure to antigen and are capable of killing some virus-infected cells and cancer cells. B and T lymphocytes appear identical and cannot be distinguished at either the light or electron microscopic level. Natural killer cells can be distinguished from B and T lymphocytes because they are generally larger and have granules in their cytoplasm. Therefore they are sometimes called *large granular lymphocytes (LGLs)*, although some cytotoxic T lymphocytes also have LGL morphology.

Natural killer cells are capable of detecting foreign cells or normal cells that fail to express normal antigens (usually because of viral infection or cancer) on their surface and can kill these cells. A single NK cell is capable of recognizing a variety of foreign cells or cells failing to express normal antigens. Because NK cells have receptors for the Fc portion of antibody molecules, they can also bind to and kill antibody-coated cells. This process is called *antibody-dependent cell-mediated cytotoxicity (ADCC)*. When NK cells detect and kill cells coated with antibody, they are sometimes referred to as *killer cells (K cells)*.

B and T lymphocytes are each capable of highly specific recognition of antigens. They are the only cells in the body capable of this extremely specific antigen recognition. They recognize antigens through antigen receptors in their cell membrane. B cells use antibody molecules as antigen receptors; T cells use T-cell receptor molecules that have structural similarities to antibody molecules. All of the antigen receptor molecules on a single B cell or T cell are essentially identical, therefore each B cell or T cell is capable of recognizing only a very restricted number of antigens.

B and T lymphocytes not only circulate through the bloodstream but also through the lymphoid tissues. Lymphocytes live for several months (and perhaps years) and are continually circulating through the blood and lymphoid tissues in search of antigens they recognize. When a lymphocyte contacts an antigen it recognizes, it initiates an antibody or cell-mediated immune response. It will take 1 to 2 weeks for an antibody or cell-mediated immune response to occur after the first exposure to antigen.

T lymphocytes can be categorized into two major types: the helper T (T_H) lymphocytes and cytotoxic T (T_C) lymphocytes. T lymphocytes can only recognize small peptide antigens that are presented on major histocompatibility complex (MHC) molecules on cells. Helper T lymphocytes secrete a variety of molecules called *cytokines* that are capable of influencing the number and activity of all of the other white blood cell types; T cytotoxic lymphocytes are capable of directly attacking and killing cells that present foreign antigens on their surface. Cells that are infected with a virus, intracellular bacterial pathogen, or that are cancerous will typically present foreign peptides on their surface and will become targets for killing by T cytotoxic cells. T cytotoxic cells are also capable of secreting cytokines that can influence other cells.

Antibodies produced by B lymphocytes and cytokines produced by T lymphocytes are capable of influencing all of the other types of leukocytes to be more effective at controlling the infectious agents or neoplastic cells that triggered the original lymphocyte response. The antibodies and cytokines produced also may be capable of directly helping to control the infectious agents or neoplastic cells without the aid of other leukocytes.

Related Topics

Phagocytic cells
Antigen receptors
T lymphocytes antigen recognition
Classes of antibody
Helper T lymphocytes
Cytokines
Natural killer cells
Hypersensitivities

Additional Reading

Abbas, A.K., Lichtman, A.H., and Pober, J.S. 1994. Chapter 2. Cells and tissues of the immune system. Cellular and Molecular Immunology, 2nd ed. W.B. Saunders, Philadelphia.

Lydyard, P. and Grossi, C. 1996. Chapter 2. Cells involved in the immune response. In Roitt, I., Brostoff, J., and Male, D. (eds.) Immunology, 4th ed. Mosby-Year Book, St. Louis.

TERMS

Cytokine	Protein molecule produced by a cell that can act on the same cell that produced it or on other cells that have receptors for the cytokine on its membrane.
Inflammation	Cellular and vascular changes that occur after tissue injury, characterized by redness, swelling, heat, and pain.
Major Histocompatibility Complex (MHC) Molecule (Types I and II)	Molecules on the membranes of cells that are highly pleiomorphic (variable) between individuals in a species and that participate in the presentation of processed peptide antigens to T lymphocytes.
Mast Cells	Cells in the tissues that are typically coated with IgE antibodies and have large granules in their cytoplasm, which contain histamine and other substances that cause dilation and increased permeability of small blood vessels.
Natural Killer Cells	A type of lymphocyte that is part of the native defense mechanisms and that can directly attack certain virally infected cells and cancer cells without previous exposure to antigen.
Thymus Gland	A primary lymphoid organ in the anterior chest cavity that is responsible for maturation of T lymphocytes.

Study Questions

1. What are the five basic types of leukocytes? Summarize key structural and functional characteristics of each type of leukocyte.
2. What is a serious side effect of drugs that suppress cell division (mitosis) in the bone marrow?
3. What are the two basic types of T lymphocytes and what are their major roles in immunity?

TOPIC 2: The Complement System

Principles

1. The complement system is an enzyme cascade system present in the plasma that can respond rapidly to attack some infectious agents and focus defense mechanisms at the site of infection. The complement cascade can be triggered by some microbial surfaces and by some antigen-antibody complexes.
2. Because the complement system involves an enzyme cascade, a small initiating signal can trigger a rapid and aggressive response. This is called *biological amplification*.
3. Activation of the complement system may help to control bacterial infection by:

- Damaging the bacterial membrane
- Attracting neutrophils to the site of infection
- Increasing blood flow to the site of infection (vasodilation)
- Facilitating leakage of plasma proteins into the site of infection (increased vascular permeability)
- Opsonizing bacteria for phagocytosis

4. Excessive activation of the complement system can lead to tissue damage.

Explanation

The complement system received its name because it complements the action of antibody in killing bacteria. Early in this century Bordet discovered that if fresh serum containing antibacterial antibody was added to bacteria it would lyse the bacteria. However, if the serum was heated to 56°C, it would not lyse the bacteria. Because the antibody activity was not destroyed by heating, he reasoned that there was another factor in the serum that was heat labile that complemented the activity of the antibody. We now know that this complementing activity was due to a group of proteins that forms a highly regulated enzyme cascade that can result in direct damage to infectious agents and the initiation of an inflammatory response to focus humoral and cellular defense mechanisms at the site of infection.

Two related, but different, enzyme cascade pathways can initiate or "activate" the complement system (Fig. 2-1). The classical pathway comprises four protein components (C1, C2, C3, and C4) and is predominantly activated by the presence of IgM or IgG antibody bound to an antigen. When the antibody molecule binds to an antigen, a conformational change occurs in the antibody molecule. The first component of complement (C1) can then bind to the changed antibody molecule. The

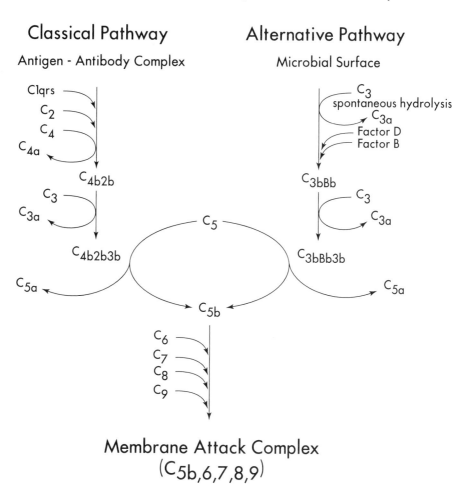

Classical Pathway

Antigen - Antibody Complex

Alternative Pathway

Microbial Surface

Membrane Attack Complex
(C5b,6,7,8,9)

Fig. 2-1   C3a, C4a, and C5a are anaphylatoxins causing mast cell degranulation, vasodilation, and greater vascular permeability. C5a is chemotactic for neutrophils.

binding of C1 to the antibody molecule causes a conformational change in C1, which converts it to an enzyme. This new C1 enzyme can then cleave multiple molecules of C2 and C4. The split pieces of C2 and C4 can combine on a cell surface and form a second enzyme (C4b,2b). This new enzyme then splits C3 into C3a and C3b. Some of the C3b can combine with the C4b,2b enzyme to create a new enzyme (C4b,2b,3b) called a *C5 convertase*, which can start the terminal pathway of complement by splitting C5 into C5a and C5b.

The alternative pathway (so named because it was described after the classical pathway and therefore was considered to be an alternative to the classical pathway) involves four proteins (factors B and D, properdin, and C3, which is also a component of the classical pathway). The alternative pathway can be activated on some microbial surfaces in the absence of antibody and therefore can play an important role in natural immunity. The key to understanding the alternative pathway is to understand that C3 in the plasma spontaneously breaks down at a slow rate into C3a and C3b. If the C3b attaches to a foreign membrane, it will be stabilized by interacting with other components of the alternative complement pathway and lead to activation of the alternative pathway and eventually the terminal complement pathway. If the spontaneously formed C3b attaches to the surface of a normal host cell, molecules on the surface of the host cell can inactivate the C3b so that it cannot start the alternative complement pathway and damage the cell. If a small amount of C3b becomes stabilized by the other components of the alternative pathway on a bacterial cell surface, then it rapidly splits more C3 and amplifies the complement reaction. Each activation pathway involves the sequential activation of three different enzymes.

Each active enzyme molecule can cleave many molecules of its substrate, thereby creating multiple active molecules of the next enzyme in the cascade. This sequential activation of enzymes gives the complement system one of its important properties: biological amplification. A small initiating stimulus (e.g., an antigen-antibody complex for the classical pathway or a suitable microbial surface for the alternative pathway) can lead to a vigorous response because it is amplified by the enzyme cascade.

All of the proteins that participate in both the classical and alternative pathways are preformed but are circulating in an inactive state, which enables the complement system to be activated very rapidly after it is initiated.

The terminal pathway (also called the *membrane attack pathway*) involves five proteins (C5, C6, C7, C8, and C9) and can be activated by either the classical or alternative pathway (see Fig. 2-1). It is initiated when C5 is split into C5a and C5b by the third enzyme (C5 convertase) formed by either the classical or alternative pathway. C5a is a small peptide that diffuses away and has many important biological activities; C5b is a larger peptide that can bind to cell surfaces immediately adjacent to where it is formed. If the C5b binds to a cell membrane, the rest of the membrane attack complex self assembles without the need for further enzyme activity. One molecule each of C6, C7, and C8 binds to the C5b molecule, then up to 15 molecules of C9 bind to this complex and form a hollow cylinder of protein inserted into the cell membrane. This effectively produces a hole in the membrane, which allows water and ions to diffuse freely into and out of the cell. If there are enough of these membrane attack complex holes in the cell, the cell will eventually rupture as a result of increased pressure from water, which is osmotically attracted into the cell.

The enzymes in the complement pathway typically cleave the substrate protein molecules into a small piece that diffuses away and a large piece that binds to surfaces very near the site of cleavage. The large pieces either contribute to forming the next enzyme in the cascade (C4b, C2b, Bb, and C3b), act as an opsonin to facilitate phagocytosis of the particle (C3b), or are the starting point for the terminal pathway (C5b). The small cleavage products that diffuse away are important initiators of the inflammatory response. C3a, C4a, and C5a are called *anaphyla-toxins* because they cause mast cell degranulation. This results in the release of histamine and other mediators, leading to vasodilation and increased vascular permeability. C5a is a strong chemoattractant for neutrophils. The end result is the diffusion of serum components (including antibody and more complement) and the egress of neutrophils into the tissues to help control the infectious agents that initiated the complement cascade.

Because the complement system can be initiated rapidly and is self-amplifying, it is very important that its activation be carefully regulated. Uncontrolled, massive activation of the complement system can cause vascular damage and initiation of the coagulation system, leading to disseminated intravascular coagulation, which is rapidly fatal. Complement system activation is regulated by the fact that the activated enzymes have a short half-life, and the cleavage products that bind to membranes have only a very brief time in which to bind or they will lose their ability to do so. There is also a group of serum proteins that help to slow complement activation by inhibiting various complement components that bind to their surface or by accelerating their decay. This helps to prevent complement damage to normal cells. However, these protective molecules can be overwhelmed by massive activation of the complement system.

In fact, it is the presence of the complement inhibitory molecules in normal host cell membranes that protect the host from the alternative complement pathway. The alternative pathway is continuously activated by spontaneous, low-level cleavage of C3 into C3a and C3b. Host cells have molecules that rapidly inactivate C3b before it can lead to amplification of the alternative pathway. Bacterial surfaces lack the inhibitory molecules, thus allowing the alternative pathway to amplify and attack the bacteria. The presence or absence of inhibitors is a crude method for the complement system to distinguish self from non-self.

The complement system is especially important for control of bacterial infections. People and animals that are deficient in key complement components (C3) are more susceptible to recurrent bacterial infections.

Additional Reading

Abbas, A.K., Lichtman, A.H., and Pober, J.S. 1994. Chapter 15. The complement system. Cellular and Molecular Immunology, 2nd ed. W.B. Saunders, Philadelphia.

Frank, M.M. and Fries, L.F. 1991. The role of complement in inflammation and phagocytosis. Immunol. Today. 12:322-326.

Morgan, B.P. and Walport, M.J. 1991. Complement deficiency and disease. Immunol. Today. 12:301-306.

Reid, K.B.M. and Day, A.J. 1989. Structure function relationships of the complement components. Immunol. Today. 12:307-311.

Walport, M. 1996. Chapter 13. Complement. In Roitt, I., Brostoff, J., and Male, D. (eds.) Immunology, 4th ed. Mosby-Year Book, St. Louis.

TERMS

Anaphylatoxins	Complement cleavage products C5a and C3a, which cause mast cell degranulation and release of histamine and other vasoactive substances.
Biological Amplification	A small stimulus is amplified into a large response, such as in an enzyme cascade system (such as complement), where one molecule of the first enzyme may activate many molecules of the next enzyme, each of which may activate many molecules of the third enzyme, etc.
Chemoattractants	Small molecules (such as some of the cleavage products of complement) that diffuse away from the site of production, forming a concentration gradient that certain cells (such as neutrophils) may follow to the source of highest concentration.
Enzyme Cascade	A series of proteins, at least some of which exist as inactive pro-enzymes. A stimulus activates the first enzyme of the cascade, which then activates the second enzyme, which can activate the third enzyme, etc.
Membrane Attack Complex	A group of complement proteins that polymerize into a cylindrical shape and insert into membranes, forming a hydrophilic channel that allows ions and water to pass through the membrane. This may lead to cell lysis.

Study Questions

1. How are each of the complement pathways activated?
2. How can a small stimulus result in extensive activation of the complement system?
3. What are the biological effects of activation of the complement system?
4. Why are exposed bacterial membranes more susceptible to damage by complement than exposed membranes of normal cells in the body?

TOPIC 3: Phagocytic Cells

Principles

1. A major immunological defense mechanism is phagocytosis, which is the process whereby particles are internalized into certain cells.
2. A bacterial infection generates chemical factors that attract large numbers of neutrophils to the site of infection in a few hours and that cause the bone marrow to rapidly release more neutrophils into the circulation.
3. Phagocytic cells are an important part of the native defense mechanisms for protecting against bacterial infection before the humoral and cell-mediated immune systems have time to react. However, phagocytic cells can be much more efficient and effective with the help of antibody and T cell cytokines.
4. Phagocytic cells kill bacteria that they have ingested (phagocytized) using the contents of their lysosomes and toxic oxygen and nitrogen metabolites generated during phagocytosis.
5. Genetic defects in phagocytic cell function or decreased phagocytic cell function caused by stress, viral infection, or drug therapy leads to increased susceptibility to bacterial infection.
6. Neutrophils recruited to inflammatory sites may contribute to tissue damage.
7. Macrophages play a very important role as antigen-presenting cells to T lymphocytes.

Explanation

Phagocytosis is the process whereby particles, such as bacteria and viruses, are taken into a cell. During phagocytosis a particle is surrounded by the membrane of a phagocytic cell, and it is internalized so that it resides in a membrane-bound vesicle (called a *phagosome*) in the cytoplasm of the phagocytic cell. Two major types of cells are considered to be professional phagocytic cells: neutrophils and the cells of the mononuclear phagocytic system (monocytes and macrophages). Neutrophils are phagocytic white blood cells that respond rapidly and aggressively to many infectious agents and other inflammatory stimuli and are short lived, whereas macrophages respond more slowly but are capable of sustained activity and killing of resistant pathogens.

Phagocytosis plays a very important role in native immunity as a first line of defense early after infection. However, phagocytic cells work much more efficiently in the presence of pathogen-specific antibody and T-cell cytokines.

For phagocytic cells to be effective, they must be targeted to the site of infection, they must ingest the infectious agent or attack infected cells, and they must have effective killing mechanisms. These activities will be explained for neutrophils, which are the prototypical phagocytic cell. Then similarities and differences with macrophages will be presented.

Neutrophils

Neutrophils are phagocytic white blood cells that are produced in the bone marrow and released in large numbers into the bloodstream. They comprise 40% to 60% of the leukocytes in the bloodstream in healthy individuals of most species, and their number increases rapidly in response to many inflammatory stimuli, especially bacterial infection. They have a half-life in the bloodstream of approximately 8 hours before migrating into the tissues. They survive for only a day or two in normal tissue and only minutes to hours at sites of inflammation. The bone marrow produces more neutrophils than any other type of white blood cell and maintains a pool of mature neutrophils to be released rapidly in response to inflammation. The body therefore makes a major commitment in bone marrow space and protein and energy utilization to produce neutrophils in large numbers. This is necessary because neutrophils are an essential first line of defense against many bacterial infections and some viral and fungal infections. When neutrophil numbers fall below 1000 per cubic millimeter in the blood, the individual is at high risk for severe bacterial infection. Some genetic defects produce specific faults in neutrophil function. Affected individuals typically have severe recurrent bacterial infections.

The neutrophil has two or three (depending on the species) types of lysosomes (also called *granules*) in its cytoplasm. Lysosomes are membrane-bound vesicles containing enzymes and cationic peptides that are important for helping the neutrophil to migrate through tissues and controlling bacterial infection. Lysosomes typically fuse with a phagosome, which is a membrane-bound vesicle containing phagocytized particles such as bacteria. This fusion of a lysosome with a phagosome containing bacteria concentrates the contents of the lysosome where they can attack the bacteria.

The neutrophil cytoplasm also contains numerous glycogen granules. Glycogen is a storage form of glucose. The neutrophil can use this stored glucose through anaerobic glycolysis as a source of energy. Because it carries its own glucose and is able to use that glucose for energy production in the absence of oxygen, the neutrophil is able to migrate into and function at sites of severe inflammation or tissue damage where there may be very low levels of blood glucose and oxygen.

To effectively control an infection, neutrophils must be able to rapidly leave the bloodstream and migrate through the tissues to sites of bacterial infection. Neutrophils normally have an adherence protein called *L-selectin* on their membrane that allows them to adhere loosely to normal capillary and small venule endothelial cells and slowly roll along the endothelium. This process is called *margination*. At any one time a large percentage of neutrophils in the blood are marginated, so that the counting of neutrophils in a peripheral blood sample underestimates the total number of neutrophils in the blood. The presence of bacteria or other inflammatory stimuli in the tissues generates various chemotactic factors such as C5a, a byproduct of complement activation. These small chemotactic stimuli diffuse from the site of production and contact endothelial cells, which causes the endothelial cells to express a new set of adherence proteins on their membrane. The chemotactic factors also contact neutrophils. The combination of the chemotactic factors contacting the neutrophils and the presence of new adherence proteins on the endothelial cells causes the neutrophil to rapidly transport new adherence proteins called *beta-integrins* to their membrane, which causes the neutrophils to stick tightly to the endothelial cells and stop rolling. Neutrophils then leave the blood vessel by diapedesis (migration between two endothelial cells) and arrive in the tissues. They then follow the gradient set up by the diffusion of chemotactic factors to the source of chemotactic factor production.

Once the neutrophils arrive at the site of bacterial infection, they must be able to phagocytize (or ingest) bacteria to kill them (Fig. 2-2). Neutrophils are capable of phagocytosing any particle that is more hydrophobic than their own membrane. Most extracellular bacterial pathogens have a hydrophilic capsule that makes them resistant to neutrophil phagocytosis. For these types of bacteria to be efficiently phagocytized, they must be coated with either antibody and/or complement components. The neutrophil membrane has receptors for the Fc portion of some classes of antibody and for the complement component C3b. The neutrophil can therefore bind to antibody or complement molecules that

OLSON LIBRARY
NORTHERN MICHIGAN UNIVERSITY
MARQUETTE, MICHIGAN 49855

Phagocytosis

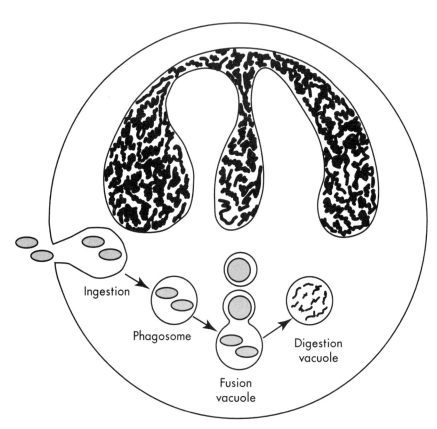

Fig. 2-2   The internalization of bacteria into a phagosome (phagocytosis) and the fusion of the phagosome with lysosomes containing antibacterial substances are necessary steps for phagocytic cells to kill bacteria.

are bound to bacterial surfaces and thereby capture and phagocytose the bacteria. A particle that is coated with antibody or complement components is said to be "opsonized" for phagocytosis. The process of phagocytosis is relatively rapid and can be completed within a few minutes.

After the neutrophil ingests the bacteria through phagocytosis, it must attempt to kill the bacteria, using two basic mechanisms. One set of mechanisms is called the *nonoxidative killing mechanisms* because it does not require the presence of oxygen to function. Its bactericidal effects are due to the actions of the enzymes and cationic antibacterial substances found within the lysosomes. After the lysosomes fuse with the phago-somes, the enzymes and cationic peptides released from the lysosomes begin to break down the bacterial cell wall and damage the bacterial cell membrane. Some bacteria have very heavy capsules that make them relatively resistant to the actions of the nonoxidative killing mechanisms. The second type of bactericidal mechanisms are referred to as the *oxidative killing mechanisms* because they require the presence of oxygen to function. The neutrophil has an oxidase enzyme that is activated during phagocytosis and generates superoxide anion, hydrogen peroxide, the hydroxyl radical, and aldehydes. All of these are capable of damaging bacteria trapped within the phagosome. This is referred to as the *oxidative burst of metabolism* because oxygen consumption by the neutrophil increases dramatically when the oxidase enzyme is activated. A very potent killing mechanism within the neutrophil involves myelo-peroxidase, an enzyme that is released into the phagosome from the lysosomes. This enzyme catalyzes a reaction between hydrogen peroxide and halide ions (iodine and chlorine), resulting in further damage to the bacteria within the phagosome. If chlorine is the halide ion involved in the reaction, hypochlorous acid is generated within the phagosome. Hypochlorous acid is the active component of chlorine bleach and is a potent bactericidal molecule.

Neutrophils may also play a role in controlling viral infections through a process called *antibody-dependent cell-mediated cytotoxicity (ADCC)*, in which neutrophils will attach to and kill a cell that is coated with antibody. If a normal cell in the body becomes infected with a virus, antibodies may form against viral proteins on the cell membrane. A neutrophil can attach to that antibody through its Fc receptors. It may then kill the cell by damaging its membrane through the actions of lysosomal enzymes and oxygen radicals.

Neutrophils from healthy individuals are normally efficient at killing bacteria. However, a number of factors are known to be capable of inhibiting or interfering with neutrophil activity. Several viral infections have been shown to inhibit neutrophil function and to predispose an individual to bacterial infections. Glucocorticoids released in response to stress and other hormones have also been shown to interfere with neutrophil function. In addition, several bacterial virulence factors are known to interfere with many aspects of neutrophil function, including inhibition of chemotaxis, phagocytosis, release of lysosomal enzymes, and oxidative metabolism. Any of these factors that inhibit neutrophil function will increase the susceptibility of an individual to infection. On the other hand, several cytokines that are released by lymphocytes and macrophages are capable of enhancing neutrophil activity and increasing the resistance of an individual to bacterial infections.

Macrophages

Macrophages are capable of nearly all of the same activities just described for neutrophils, but they conduct these activities differently. Macrophages live much longer than do neutrophils; further, they can repair their own membranes and replenish their enzymes and lysosomes. They are much slower to arrive at sites of infection than are neutrophils, but they can survive longer at the site and are able to kill some pathogens that are resistant to killing by neutrophils. This is especially true if the macrophages have been activated by T lymphocyte-derived cytokines. If a lesion is characterized by the infiltration of neutrophils, it is classified as an acute inflammatory reaction. If it is characterized by the infiltration of mononuclear cells (macrophages and lymphocytes), it is classified as a chronic inflammatory reaction.

Macrophages are also important in the immune response because they release several cytokines and other molecules that influence other aspects of the immune system. They are especially active at releasing proinflammatory cytokines early in infection that induce fever, malaise, and other symptoms associated with infection. Some of the factors released by macrophages are important for facilitating wound healing.

In addition to acting as a phagocytic cell for controlling infection, macrophages also play a very important role in processing and presenting antigens to T helper lymphocytes. This is essential for induction of a cell-mediated immune response.

Related Topics

T lymphocyte antigen recognition
Cytokines
Leukocyte trafficking
The acute phase response

Additional Reading

Densen, P., Clark, R.A., and Nauseef, W.M. 1995. Chapter 7. Granulocytic phagocytes. In Mandell, G.L., Bennett, J.E., and Dolin, R. (eds.) Principles and Practice of Infectious Diseases. Churchill Livingstone, New York.

Domachowske, J.B. and Malech, H.L. 1996. Chapter 25. Phagocytes. In Rich R.R. (ed.) Clinical Immunology: Principles and Practice. Mosby-Year Book, St. Louis.

Van Furth, R. 1992. Mononuclear phagocyte system. In Roitt, I.M. and Delves, P.J. (eds.) Encyclopedia of Immunology. Academic Press, San Diego.

TERMS

Antibody-dependent Cell-mediated Cytotoxicity (ADCC)	The destruction of antibody-coated target cells by cells such as neutrophils, macrophages, eosinophils, or killer lymphocytes, which can bind to the Fc portion of the antibody molecules and thereby attack the target cell.
Cationic Antibacterial Peptides	Peptides with a positive net charge that can polymerize and insert into some bacterial cell membranes to form pores that damage or kill the bacteria.
Degranulation	The process whereby a phagosome fuses with a lysosome to expose particles in the phagosome to the antimicrobial substances in the lysosome.
Diapedesis	The process by which a white blood cell leaves the bloodstream by passing between two endothelial cells.
Lysosome	Membrane-bound vesicle in phagocytic cells that contains enzymes, cationic proteins, and other substances to help kill and degrade microorganisms.
Opsonization	The process whereby a particle is coated with antibody and/or complement to facilitate phagocytosis.
Phagosome	Membrane-bound vesicle in the cytoplasm of a phagocytic cell that contains the phagocytosed particle.

Study Questions

1. What mechanisms allow neutrophils to leave the vascular system and enter the tissues at sites of infection?
2. What factors can opsonize particles to facilitate phagocytosis?
3. How does a phagocytic cell kill bacteria?
4. How can phagocytic cells help to control viral infections?
5. What are some factors or conditions that will suppress phagocytic cell function and lead to increased susceptibility to bacterial infection?

TOPIC 4: The Lymphoid System

Principles

1. Lymphocytes that react with self antigens are eliminated during development in primary lymphoid tissues.
2. Organized secondary lymphoid tissues (e.g., lymph nodes and spleen) are sites where antigens are collected and presented to lymphocytes.
3. Lymphocytes circulate between blood and lymphoid tissues to optimize their chances for encountering antigens.

Explanation

The lymphoid system of the body is a collection of organs and tissues involved in the production and maturation of lymphocytes and in the generation of antigen-specific immune responses. These sites can be divided into primary and secondary lymphoid tissues. Primary lymphoid tissues are responsible for the proliferation and maturation of lymphocytes. Secondary lymphoid tissues, which are seeded with lymphocytes from primary tissues, provide a suitable environment for the interaction of antigens, antigen-presenting cells, and lymphocytes to initiate immune responses.

Lymphocytes, like other types of blood cells, are generated in early embryos first by the primitive omentum and then by the yolk sac and fetal liver. Later in fetal life, and through adult life, this function is performed almost exclusively by the bone marrow. The lymphocytes that are released by these tissues are still immature and nonfunctional; they migrate in the blood to the primary lymphoid organs for further maturation.

Within primary lymphoid tissues, immature lymphocytes undergo several selection processes that determine whether an individual lymphocyte will mature or die. Most of the lymphocytes that migrate to primary lymphoid organs will die there. Lymphocytes that cannot recognize antigens or those that recognize the host's own tissue antigens are largely eliminated in this process. A small percentage of incoming lymphocytes is allowed to mature; these are the lymphocytes that recognize foreign antigens. Lymphocytes that are selected to mature proliferate to form clones of identical cells, thus increasing the populations of foreign antigen-specific lymphocytes. They also undergo a series of changes in the types and quantities of receptor molecules that they express (display) on their cell surfaces. Proper receptor expression is important because all of a lymphocyte's immunological functions involve specific receptor interactions with soluble molecules or other cell-bound receptors. When lymphocytes are released from primary lymphoid tissues, they are mature, albeit virginal, functional cells.

The thymus serves as a primary lymphoid organ in mammals and birds. Lymphocytes that mature within the thymus are called *T-,* or *thymus-derived, lymphocytes,* and they are the lymphocytes that mediate cell-mediated immune responses. The thymus is a lobular mass of tissue located in the anterior thorax and/or neck. The thymus is organized into an outer cortex and an inner medulla. The most immature lymphocytes are located in the cortex, and as they mature, they migrate toward the medulla. From the medulla, mature lymphocytes are released into the blood or lymph.

The primary lymphoid organ for the maturation of antibody-producing lymphocytes varies among animal species. In birds the organ is the bursa of Fabricius, which forms a pouch adjacent to the cloaca. Because the bursa of Fabricius was the first primary lymphoid organ described for the maturation of antibody-producing lymphocytes, such lymphocytes are also called *B-,* or *bursal-derived, lymphocytes.* Mammals have no lymphoid tissue that is structurally equivalent to the bursa. In humans and most domesticated mammals, the bone marrow serves as the primary lymphoid organ for B cells. Ruminant animals (e.g., cattle, sheep, goats) possess a specialized form of intestinal lymph nodes (ileocecal Peyer's patches), where B lymphocytes undergo maturation. The bursa of Fabricius and ileocecal Peyer's patches are also compartmentalized into cortical and medullary regions.

Primary lymphoid organs arise early in fetal life. They are most prominent in young, healthy animals and shrink in size after sexual maturity. The thymus, ileocecal Peyer's patches, and bursa of Fabricius atrophy, often becoming small remnants of tissue in elderly individuals. The functional capacity of bone marrow also shrinks with age as the active cellular components are replaced by fat cells. The decreasing size and function of primary lymphoid tissues in aged individuals has been implicated as a contributory factor in immune senescence, the age-related decline in immune function. However, even aged primary lymphoid tissues do retain some function and continue to supply lymphocytes for secondary tissues throughout life.

After lymphocytes leave the primary lymphoid organs, they migrate to secondary lymphoid tissues. Secondary lymphoid tissues arise late in fetal life, but they persist throughout the life of the individual. Secondary lymphoid tissues include lymph nodes and the spleen, as well as microscopic lymphoid nodules scattered throughout mucosal sites of the body (e.g., intestine, respiratory tract, reproductive tract).

Lymphocytes may enter lymph nodes via the blood or the lymph. Small veins within lymph nodes called *high endothelial venules* are lined by specialized endothelial cells that allow naive lymphocytes to exit the blood rapidly and efficiently and enter the lymph node tissue. About 90% of the lymphocytes that enter lymph node tissue are derived from the blood. The rest of the lymphocytes are derived from lymph, which is a lymphocyte-rich fluid that is transported in a series of vessels called the *lymphatic system*. Lymph fluid originates in the tissues as a transudate from plasma.

Lymphatic vessels are similar to blood vessels except that they do not form a complete (closed) system. Most tissues are drained by lymphatic vessels, as well as veins, and the flow of lymph serves as an efficient means of transporting antigens and lymphocytes from various tissues to lymph nodes, which are located along the course of lymphatic vessels. Lymphatic vessels eventually empty into the thoracic duct, the largest lymph vessel. The thoracic duct then empties into a large vein near the heart. Thus, lymphocytes migrate freely between the blood and lymph.

Lymph nodes serve as a collecting point for antigens and lympho-cytes. They enhance antigen/lymphocyte interactions by providing the proper environment in which lymphocytes can recognize their comple-mentary antigens and be activated. Lymph nodes contain large numbers of macrophages and dendritic cells, which serve as antigen presenting cells and provide necessary costimulatory signals for lymphocyte activa-tion. Lymph nodes also can control the rate of lymphocyte migration through the node. If the lymph node becomes inflamed or infected, lymphocytes are held for longer periods within the lymph node tissue, which enhances the probability that lymphocytes will encounter their complementary antigen. Once lymphocytes have been activated within the lymph node, many of them migrate to the tissues from which the inciting foreign antigen was derived, thus localizing immune defenses at the inflamed/infected site.

Lymph nodes of humans and most animal species are organized into an outer cortex and inner medulla (Fig. 2-3). The exception is in pigs and related species, where the orientation is reversed. B lymphocytes are concen-trated in the outer cortex and medulla. The paracortical region, located between the cortex and medulla, is rich in T lymphocytes. Lymphocytes in the cortex are organized into clusters or nodules. When lymphocytes in these nodules are stimulated by antigen, there is intense proliferation within the nodules; the active nodules are called *germinal centers*.

The spleen serves as a secondary lymphoid tissue in a manner similar to lymph nodes except that the spleen does not receive lymphatic drainage. It serves as a filter for the blood, and blood-borne antigens are trapped within the spleen. The spleen is arranged into red pulp, where the blood-filtering functions are performed, and the white pulp, where the spleen's immunological functions take place (Fig. 2-4). Lymphocytes are concentrated around small arteries (arterioles) and form periarteriolar lymphoid sheaths. The sheaths are rich in T lymphocytes, but they also contain scattered nodules of B cells.

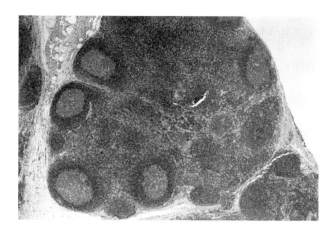

Fig. 2-3 Human lymph node showing cortex and medullary areas and germinal centers. (From Rich, R.R. [ed.] 1996. Clinical Immunology: Principles and Practice. Mosby-Year Book, St. Louis.)

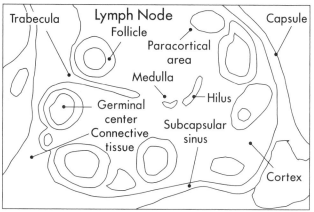

The bone marrow acts as a secondary lymphoid tissue, as well as a primary lymphoid tissue. It contains many monocytes and macrophages that can scavenge antigen and present it to lymphocytes. The bone marrow is an important site of antibody production in immune animals undergoing memory responses. There is also evidence that the bursa of Fabricius can trap and present certain antigens to lymphocytes residing there.

Numerous scattered foci of lymphoid tissue are located in submucosal tissues. These sites are often known by acronyms, such as GALT (gut-associated lymphoid tissue) or BALT (bronchus-associated lymphoid tissue). Collectively they are sometimes called MALT (mucosal-associated lymphoid tissue). These sites play important roles in local immunity at body surfaces, and their importance has been increasingly appreciated by immunologists in recent years. Resting lymphocytes may be stimulated by antigen within MALT, producing local immunity that is independent of systemic responses.

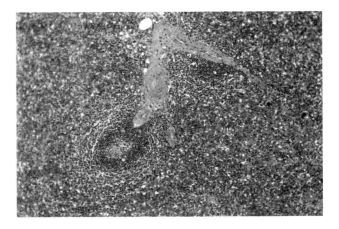

Fig. 2-4   Human spleen showing a periarteriolar lymphoid sheath and germinal center. (From Rich, R.R. [ed.] 1996. Clinical Immunology: Principles and Practice. Mosby-Year Book, St. Louis.)

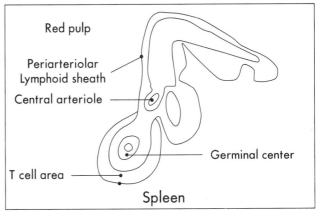

Related Topics

T lymphocyte antigen recognition
Costimulatory signals for lymphocytes
Recognition of self vs. non-self
Mucosal immunity

Additional Reading

Lewis, D. and Harriman, G.R. 1996. Chapter 2. Cells and tissues of the immune system. In Rich, R.R. (ed.) Clinical Immunology: Principles and Practice. Mosby-Year Book, St. Louis.
Tizard, I. 1996. Chapter 8. The organs of the immune system. In Veterinary Immunology: An Introduction, 5th ed. W.B. Saunders, Philadelphia.

TERMS

High Endothelial Venules	Small veins with specialized lining (endothelium) characterized by tall columnar cells that allow passage of lymphocytes out of the vascular system into underlying lymphoid tissue.
Lymph	Lymphocyte-rich fluid (transudate) that drains from tissue spaces into the lymphatic system.
Lymphatic System	Series of lymph vessels, similar to blood vessels, that carry lymph from tissues back to the bloodstream. Unlike the cardiovascular system, the lymphatic system is not closed; it empties into a series of larger vessels, ending with the thoracic duct, which empties into a blood vessel near the heart.
Mucosal-associated Lymphoid Tissue (MALT)	Scattered foci of lymphoid tissue associated with mucosal sites, such as the intestine, respiratory tract, and reproductive tract.
Primary Lymphoid Tissue	Lymphoid tissues where lymphocytes are selectively eliminated or allowed to mature for release into circulation based on their antigen reactivity. Includes the thymus, bone marrow, bursa of Fabricius (birds), and ileocecal lymph nodes (ruminants).
Secondary Lymphoid Tissue	Lymphoid tissues where mature lymphocytes encounter antigen and proliferate in response to antigenic stimulation. Includes most lymph nodes throughout the body, the spleen, and mucosal-associated lymphoid tissue.

Study Questions

1. What are the major functions of primary lymphoid tissues? Secondary lymphoid tissues?
2. What is the route that lymphocytes use to circulate throughout the body?
3. How does lymphocyte circulation serve to enhance the ability of the immune system to fight infection?

Antigen Recognition

Acquired immunity requires extremely precise recognition of foreign invaders and abnormal cells. This is needed so that the potent killing mechanisms of the immune system will be unleashed rapidly on foreign invaders and to prevent these killing mechanisms from being activated against normal cells and tissues. The specific recognition of antigen also is needed to enable the immune system to recognize and remember pathogens it has encountered previously, so that it can more rapidly and aggressively attack these pathogens when they are encountered again.

Both B lymphocytes, which are responsible for humoral immunity (antibodies), and T lymphocytes, which are responsible for cell-mediated immunity, use antigen receptors on their surface that specifically recognize only small portions of foreign molecules on a pathogen. The B and T cell populations each are capable of recognizing a great diversity of foreign molecules. To understand the immune response, it is essential to understand how B and T cells recognize antigens. It is also important to understand how B and T cell populations are able to generate the great diversity of antigen recognition molecules that allow them to recognize an almost unlimited array of foreign molecules.

List of Principles

Antigen Receptors Lymphocytes recognize specific antigens through specialized receptors on their cell surfaces.

B lymphocytes use a sample of the type of antibody molecules they are capable of secreting as membrane-bound receptors for antigens.

Continued

List of Principles — cont'd

T lymphocytes detect specific antigens in the environment by a membrane-bound receptor that is similar to, but distinct from, antibody.

Antigen receptors for B and T lymphocytes contain auxiliary protein chains to stabilize bonds between receptor and antigen and to transmit signals to the interior of the cell.

Antigen-Receptor Interaction

B and T lymphocytes recognize antigen by forming noncovalent bonds of high affinity to portions of molecules a few amino acids in size.

The closeness of fit and the distribution of positive and negative charges between the three-dimensional structures of antigen and receptor determine whether bonds of high affinity may form between molecules.

It is possible for a lymphocyte to recognize a group of related antigens if the structure of the antigens at the recognition sites is similar.

Antigen Receptor Diversity

The tremendous diversity and specificity of immune recognition by both B and T lymphocytes are accomplished during development through modification of the genes that encode antigen receptors.

Genetic modification of antigen receptor genes is random.

Diversity at each of the critical steps in the modification process allows for the generation of millions of different antigen receptors.

Clonal Development of Lymphocytes

B and T lymphocytes divide to produce large clones (approximately 10^9 in mammals).

Lymphocytes of the same clone recognize exactly the same antigens.

Clonal expansion after exposure to an antigen is a means of increasing the number of lymphocytes that are reactive against that antigen.

Increased numbers of cells in the clones that recognize an antigen is the basis for immunological memory.

T Lymphocyte Antigen Recognition

T lymphocytes are capable only of recognizing small pieces of antigen that have been processed and presented by genetically matched antigen-presenting cells.

■ List of Principles — cont'd ■

Antigen-presenting cells degrade whole antigens into small fragments that lymphocytes can recognize.

Antigen-presenting cells combine antigen fragments with major histocompatibility complex (MHC) molecules for presentation to T lymphocytes.

T lymphocytes only recognize antigens that are presented on cells possessing MHC molecules identical to those of the lymphocyte.

There is great genetic diversity of MHC molecules among individuals of the same species.

Costimulatory Signals for Lymphocytes

Both B and T lymphocytes must recognize antigen and receive costimulatory signals to produce an immune response.

The nature of costimulatory signals influences the type of immune response that is generated.

Requirements for costimulation are reduced in previously activated lymphocytes.

Helper T lymphocytes that recognize antigen are an important source of costimulatory signals for B lymphocytes.

Superantigens

Superantigens from bacteria and viruses are antigens that activate multiple clones of T lymphocytes.

Superantigens are not recognized by T lymphocytes in the same manner as conventional antigens.

Large-scale immune activation by superantigens can cause severe clinical disease.

Superantigens cross-link MHC and T-cell receptor molecules by binding to each of them outside of the normal antigen-binding site.

Recognition of Self vs. Non-Self

The immune system does not normally react to self antigens. This is known as tolerance.

The immune system learns to distinguish self from non-self primarily during fetal development.

The process of thymic selection eliminates T lymphocytes that recognize self.

Non-self antigens residing within an individual before T and B lymphocytes mature in fetal development are treated as self antigens by the developing immune system.

Continued

━━━━━━━━━━ **List of Principles — cont'd** ━━━━━━━━━━

Tolerance   An individual's immune system may become tolerant of specific antigens. Tolerance may be temporary or long-lived.

Tolerance may be induced centrally (within primary lymphoid tissues during lymphocyte development) or at peripheral sites.

Antigens residing in immune-privileged sites are relatively protected from immune attack even though the immune system may attack the same antigens if located elsewhere in the body.

Lack of immune response through tolerance is a distinct phenomenon from lack of response caused by immunodeficiency.

TOPIC 1: Antigen Receptors

Principles

1. Lymphocytes recognize specific antigens through specialized receptors on their cell surfaces.
2. B lymphocytes use a sample of the type of antibody molecules they are capable of secreting as membrane-bound receptors for antigens.
3. T lymphocytes detect specific antigens in the environment by a membrane-bound receptor that is similar to, but distinct from, antibody.
4. Antigen receptors for B and T lymphocytes contain auxiliary protein chains to stabilize bonds between receptor and antigen and to transmit signals to the interior of the cell.

Explanation

The specificity of the immune system of higher vertebrates relies on the ability of lymphocytes to differentiate among the antigens in their environment and to react against those antigens that are foreign. Individual animals are able to discriminate among millions of different antigens because they possess millions of different lymphocytes, each developed to recognize and react to antigens that are complementary to (bind to) its own antigen receptor. The antigen specificity of an individual lymphocyte is determined by the type of antigen receptor molecules that are found on the cell's surface. All of the antigen receptors on an individual lymphocyte are identical, but lymphocytes with differing antigenic specificities have unique receptors. Antigen receptor molecules on the surface membrane of the lymphocyte continually monitor the environment around the lymphocyte and send biochemical signals to the lymphocyte nucleus when an antigen molecule with a shape and charge distribution complementary to the receptor molecule binds to the receptor.

Antigen receptors for T lymphocytes, also called *T-cell receptors (TCRs),* are composed of a complex of molecules (Fig. 3-1). There are two major classes of TCRs: alpha-beta (α/β) and gamma-delta (γ/δ). These class designations refer to the types of protein chains that form the antigen-binding portion of the TCR. Lymphocytes expressing α/β TCRs are the most common, and most of our knowledge about antigen recognition is based on studies of α/β T cells. However, interest in γ/δ cells, which may play a role in immunity at mucosal surfaces, has increased in recent years.

In addition to the antigen-binding protein chains, the TCR also contains coreceptor proteins, CD4 or CD8. T lymphocytes recognize antigen that forms a complex with major histocompatibility complex (MHC) molecules on antigen-presenting cells. The coreceptor proteins bind to the MHC molecule at a site away from where the antigen is located. Coreceptor proteins provide stabilization to the fragile bond

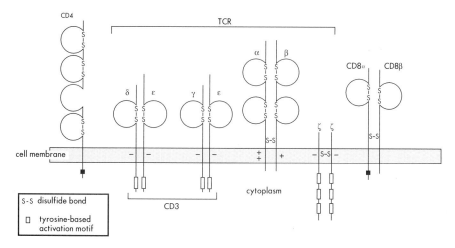

Fig. 3-1 Schematic representation of the human TCR and CD4 and CD8 coreceptors. Immunoglobulin-like regions are represented by loops. CD3 and ζ (zeta) chains make up the invariant complex; note that these proteins contain tails that extend into the cytoplasm for signaling across the cell membrane. Most mature lymphocytes express either CD4 or CD8, and not both. (Modified from Rich, R.R. [ed.] 1996. Clinical Immunology: Principles and Practice. Mosby-Year Book, St. Louis.)

between antigen/MHC complexes and the lymphocyte, increasing binding affinity up to 100-fold. Coreceptors also may influence the type of stimulatory signal that is transmitted through the TCR because expression of CD4 or CD8 is closely associated with subsequent effector functions of the stimulated lymphocyte. (CD4+ lymphocytes usually provide helper functions, and CD8+ lymphocytes are usually cytotoxic to cells harboring foreign antigens.) The nature of the qualitative differences in the stimulatory signals generated by CD4+ and CD8+ lymphocytes is yet unclear. However, activation of lymphocytes requires successful coreceptor binding; in fact, binding of antigen without coreceptor binding can actually inhibit the ability of the lymphocyte to respond to subsequent antigenic stimulation.

The TCR also contains a group of proteins called the invariant CD3 complex, so named because the proteins in this complex are highly similar among lymphocytes of different animal species. The invariant CD3 complex is involved in transmitting the signals generated on the extracellular portion of the TCR to the interior of the lymphocyte. It is also involved in the reception of costimulatory signals from the antigen-presenting cell. The biochemical reactions that are involved in transmitting activation signals to the lymphocyte are very complex and only partially understood. However, signal transduction often occurs through the phosphorylation of specific amino acids of cell proteins mediated through enzymes of the kinase family.

Antigen receptors of B lymphocytes are also composed of a complex of proteins (Fig. 3-2). The core molecule of the B-cell receptor is an antibody molecule. Membrane-bound antibodies have the same antigen specificity as the antibodies that are secreted by that particular lymphocyte. They are usually of the same isotype as that secreted by the cell, except for virgin cells, which often express IgD on their surfaces even though they do not release IgD antibodies into the extracellular environment. They are bound to the surface of the lymphocyte by their Fc segments (see topic on classes of antibody for discussion of antibody structure) so that their antigen-binding (Fab) segments are exposed to the extracellular environment.

B-cell receptors also appear to have a coreceptor, which is formed by the combination of two proteins, CD19 and CD21. Because B lymphocytes can recognize particulate antigen in the absence of major histocompatibility molecules, the function of the coreceptor is less clear. However, because CD21 can bind to complement, the coreceptor may serve to stabilize interactions with antigens that have complement bound to their surfaces.

B-cell receptors also have invariant complexes to mediate signal transduction to the interior of the lymphocyte. The invariant complex of

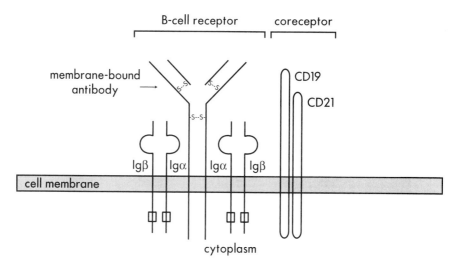

Fig. 3-2 B-cell antigen receptor structure.

the B lymphocyte is composed of two proteins, Igα and Igβ. The biochemical reactions that mediate signal transduction are probably similar to those used by T lymphocytes.

The number of antigen receptors on the surface of a lymphocyte may vary throughout the life of a cell. Resting, unstimulated lymphocytes have fewer receptors than do activated lymphocytes. Lymphocytes in close proximity to activated lymphocytes may also have increased receptor densities because cytokines, such as interleukin-2 or gamma-interferon, produced by the activated cells can induce neighboring lymphocytes to express more antigen receptors on their surfaces. Lymphocytes that express many antigen receptors are more likely to bind successfully with, and be activated by, small concentrations of antigen than are lymphocytes with few antigen receptors, so increasing receptor density is a mechanism whereby the immune system can become more sensitive to the presence of antigens.

Related Topics

Antigen receptor diversity
T lymphocyte antigen recognition
Costimulatory signals for lymphocytes
Classes of antibody
Cytokines
Intraepithelial lymphocytes

Additional Reading

Chan, A.C., Desai, D.M., and Weiss, A. 1994. The role of protein tyrosine kinases and protein tyrosine phosphatases in T cell antigen receptor signal transduction. Annu. Rev. Immunol. 12:555-592.

Janeway, C.A. Jr. 1992. The T cell receptor as a multicomponent signalling machine: CD4/CD8 coreceptors and CD45 in T cell activation. Annu. Rev. Immunol. 10:645-674.

Marrack, P. and Kappler, J. 1986. The T cell and its receptor. Sci. Am. 254:36-45.

Weiss, A. and Littman, D.R. 1994. Signal transduction by lymphocyte antigen receptors. Cell. 76:263-274.

TERMS:

B-cell Receptor (BCR)	The molecular structure on the surface of a B lymphocyte through which the lymphocyte recognizes antigen. The main structure is an immunoglobulin (antibody) molecule, similar to the antibodies that the cell secretes. Additional proteins aid in transmission of activation signals to the cell interior.
T-cell Coreceptor	The molecule (CD4 or CD8) that stabilizes the bond between the TCR and antigen.
T-cell Receptor (TCR)	The molecular structure on the surface of a T lymphocyte through which the lymphocyte recognizes antigen. The TCR is composed of an immunoglobulin-like structure that binds with the antigen and several other proteins that transmit activation signals to the interior of the cell. Two types of TCRs have been identified: α/β TCRs, which are the most common, and γ/δ TCRs.

Study Questions

1. What are the major characteristics of the antigen receptor molecules used by B and T lymphocytes?
2. What are coreceptor molecules on B and T cells, and what are their functions?
3. What are the invariant complex molecules on B and T cells, and what are their functions?

TOPIC 2: Antigen-Receptor Interaction

Principles

1. B and T lymphocytes recognize antigen by forming noncovalent bonds of high affinity to portions of molecules a few amino acids in size.
2. The closeness of fit and the distribution of positive and negative charges between the three-dimensional structures of antigen and receptor determine whether bonds of high affinity may form between molecules.
3. It is possible for a lymphocyte to recognize a group of related antigens if the structure of the antigens at the recognition sites is similar.

Explanation

A key feature of the immune system of higher vertebrates is the ability to initiate immune responses that are directed specifically against foreign antigens. This ability allows the immune system to exert potent, lethal effects on foreign antigens without causing undue damage to the normal host tissues surrounding the antigen. To achieve this selectivity, the immune system must discriminate among individual antigens and activate only those lymphocytes that are programmed to react against the encountered antigen. Lymphocytes that can react against a particular antigen have a receptor structure that has a type of "mirror image" to the structure of the antigen. Consequently, when a lymphocyte comes into contact with its complementary antigen, there is a very close structural fit between the receptor and antigen. This close fit provides a signal necessary to activate the lymphocyte.

The parts of the receptor protein and antigen that come into close approximation during the antigen recognition process are actually very small segments of the overall receptor and antigen molecules. Multiple segments of a few amino acids in length may be involved. The segments may be located at separate sites along the amino acid chains of the molecules, but the segments are juxtaposed when the molecules are folded into their functional three-dimensional structures (Fig. 3-3). The binding site of the antigen is called an *epitope*. The complementary structure on the receptor that binds to the epitope is called a *paratope*.

A complex antigen may have several different epitopes on different parts of its overall structure that can be recognized by lymphocytes. Therefore, one antigen may activate several different clones of lymphocytes. If several clones are activated, the immune response may be strengthened because the resultant antibodies and cell-mediated processes will be

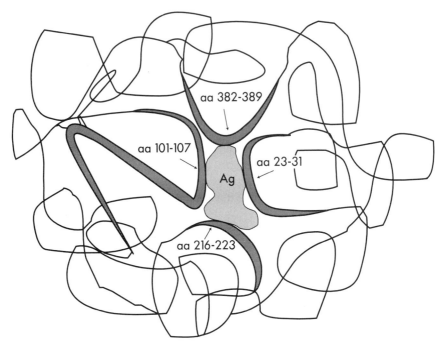

Fig. 3-3   Representative three-dimensional structure of antigen/antibody interaction. The protein chains of an antibody form three-dimensional globular structures; multiple short stretches of amino acids (aa) bind to the antigen. The antigen contact points may be widely separated on the linear antibody protein, but they are brought into approximation when the protein folds into its functional conformation.

directed against multiple parts of the antigen, some of which are more vulnerable than others to inactivation and/or elimination of the antigen.

When a lymphocyte receptor binds to its complementary antigen, the two molecules are not irreversibly attached to each other. Rather, they are held together by forces that are generated when two molecules come into close contact with each other (i.e., noncovalent forces). These forces include hydrogen bonds, electrostatic attraction between oppositely charged amino acids, and the attraction that occurs when two molecules come into such close contact that water molecules between them are excluded. The strength of all of these forces is dependent on the closeness of the contact between two molecules. If two molecules cannot come into close contact because their structures are not highly complementary, the resultant forces are too weak to bind the molecules together. The strength of the noncovalent binding, which is proportional to the degree of fit between antigen and lymphocyte receptor, is called *binding affinity*. An activation signal is generated within a lymphocyte when an antigen binds with high affinity to its receptors. Various costimulatory signals are needed to activate the lymphocyte fully.

The pairing of one lymphocyte specificity with one complementary antigen is not absolute. Because there are millions of antigens in the host's environment, some similarities in structure are bound to exist between some of them. If an antigen that is structurally related to the complementary antigen of a particular lymphocyte comes into contact with that lymphocyte, some degree of antigen binding may take place. In many instances, the fit between antigen and receptor is poor enough that the binding affinity is below the threshold needed to activate the lymphocyte. In other cases, though, the lymphocyte may be activated by the related antigen, a phenomenon called *cross-reactivity.*

Cross-reactivity has been used clinically to immunize humans and animals against diseases for which direct vaccination is undesirable or ineffective. For example, in the late 1700s, Jenner used the cowpox virus to immunize people against smallpox, a related lethal virus. If people contracted smallpox without prior exposure to cowpox, many of them died. However, Jenner discovered that people who had recovered from cowpox, which causes mild skin infections in humans, were protected against subsequent exposure to smallpox virus. We now know that the reason this vaccination strategy worked was because lymphocytes that were activated by the cowpox virus generated memory lymphocytes that could be reactivated by either cowpox or smallpox viruses to generate a strong, quick immune response that would eliminate either virus.

Related Topic

Costimulatory signals for lymphocytes

Additional Readings

Ashwell, J.D. and Weissman, A.M. 1996. Chapter 5. T-cell receptor genes, gene products, and coreceptors. In Rich, R.R. (ed.) Clinical Immunology: Principles and Practice. Mosby-Year Book, St. Louis.
Voet, D. and Voet, J.G. 1995. Chapter 7. Three-dimensional structures of proteins. Biochemistry. 2nd ed. J. Wiley and Sons, New York.

TERM:

Epitope
The site on an antigen that is recognized by lymphocytes. An antigen may possess many epitopes within its structure. Epitopes consist of only a few amino acids, and they may be

dependent on the three-dimensional folding of the antigen for their structure.

Study Questions

1. What types of chemical bonds hold antigens and antigen-receptor molecules (antibody or T-cell receptors) together?
2. Name a type of chemical bond that is never involved in antigen-antigen receptor binding.
3. Approximately how large is an epitope on an antigen that an antigen receptor molecule recognizes?
4. What determines the affinity of binding between antigens and antigen receptor molecules?

TOPIC 3: Antigen Receptor Diversity

Principles

1. The tremendous diversity and specificity of immune recognition by both B and T lymphocytes are accomplished during development through modification of the genes that encode antigen receptors.
2. Genetic modification of antigen receptor genes is random.
3. Diversity at each of the critical steps in the modification process allows for the generation of millions of different antigen receptors.

Explanation

Lymphocyte precursors, when they are first produced in the thymus or bone marrow, are alike in genetic composition within an individual animal or human being. If mature lymphocytes were derived in an identical manner from these precursors, all lymphocytes would produce identical receptor proteins (antibodies or T-cell receptors for B and T lymphocytes, respectively) that would recognize the same antigen. However, there are many different antigens in an animal's environment, and the immune system must be able to recognize nearly all of them that are foreign. Therefore, the immune system needs lymphocytes with many different antigenic specificities. To achieve this necessary diversity, individual lymphocyte precursors undergo a maturation process whereby their genetic compositions are altered so that they encode unique receptor proteins. Lymphocytes possessing different receptors recognize and respond to different antigens.

There are four basic mechanisms by which diverse receptor genes may be produced during lymphocyte maturation: genetic rearrangement, junctional diversity, somatic mutation, and combinatorial diversity (Fig. 3-4).

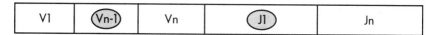

Germline DNA contains many alleles of V and J gene segments.
One allele of each segment is selected for use.

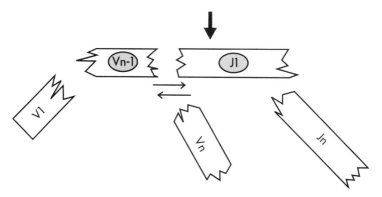

Extra DNA is excised and selected segments are brought together.

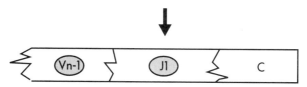

Gene segments are joined with one another and with
a constant (C) segment to form a functional receptor gene.
(Joining may also occur at the RNA level.)

Genes may undergo further mutation at specific base pairs.

Fig. 3-4   Generation of antigen receptor diversity (immunoglobulin light chain).

Genetic rearrangement

Antigen receptor proteins are encoded on several scattered gene segments that must be brought into juxtaposition as one continuous stretch of DNA before they are functional. Gene segments for two different genes must rearrange properly before a functional receptor can be produced because antigen receptors are composed of two proteins. The genes for the light chain of the B-cell receptor and the alpha chain of the T-cell receptor have three segments: V, J, and C. The genes for the heavy chain of the B-cell receptor and the beta chain of the T-cell receptor possess four segments: V, D, J, and C. In their native unarranged (germline) form, chromosomes possess the genetic information for many versions of each of the V, D, and J segments. There may be 4 to 200 versions, depending on the segment type and the species of animal involved. However, only one version of each segment is incorporated into the final gene sequence. During lymphocyte development, one version of each of the V, D, and J segments is selected, and the DNA encoding the remaining versions is eliminated or not used. The selected segments are then joined with one another and with the invariant C (constant) segment to form antigen receptor genes. Diversity among lymphocyte receptors is generated by the random selection of gene segments.

Junctional diversity

The selected gene segments must be joined together to form one continuous length of DNA. Although there are preferred nucleotide sequences at the ends of each gene segment where joining is most likely to occur, the junctional sites are not absolute. The actual junctional site can vary by several nucleotide pairs. The addition or deletion of even one nucleotide pair in the final gene can alter the amino acid sequence of the protein that is produced from that gene. Thus, additional receptor diversity is generated by the relative laxity in gene segment junctional sites.

Somatic mutation

The rearranged, joined genes that encode antigen receptor proteins are subject to errors when chromosomes are duplicated as cells divide. They also are subject to errors when damaged DNA is repaired. Point mutations, which result in a change in the identity of one nucleotide, are common within antigen receptor genes. If a nucleotide substitution alters the identity of an amino acid that is incorporated into an antigen receptor protein, the specificity of the overall antigen receptor could be altered. Somatic mutations do contribute to the generation of antigenic diversity in developing virgin lymphocyte populations, but the impact of somatic mutations on the generation of receptor diversity is probably greatest during affinity maturation of antibody responses.

Combinatorial diversity

Because antigen receptors are composed of two separate protein chains, additional receptor diversity is generated when these two chains combine. Each protein is encoded by a separate gene and synthesized independently of the other within the lymphocyte. Therefore it is possible, for example, for two lymphocytes that produce identical heavy chains to produce unique light chains. The specificity of the antigen receptors of these two lymphocytes would be different from each other because antigens bind in three-dimensional clefts formed by the physical interactions of both protein chains. The uniqueness of the light chains would alter the conformation of the antigen-binding cleft.

The factors that stimulate individual lymphocyte precursors to undergo unique genetic modifications that affect antigen recognition are incompletely understood. However, the process is carefully controlled in that lymphocytes that fail to undergo successful genetic modifications and do not proliferate will undergo apoptosis (programmed cell death) in the thymus or bone marrow. Each modification of DNA structure has the potential to generate a gene sequence that encodes a functional protein or to generate a nonsense sequence. Only those lymphocytes with functional gene sequences continue to develop, and this subset constitutes a very small percentage of the original pool of lymphocyte precursors. Furthermore, only a very small portion of the receptor protein determines antigen specificity; genetic modifications must occur in the proper location to affect the scope of immune recognition. Finally, the immune system then determines which lymphocytes are reactive against self antigens (i.e., antigens normally present in the body) and eliminates them. Despite the great odds against generating a lymphocyte with a unique specificity, it is estimated that mammals generate lymphocytes with several million different antigenic specificities.

Related Topics

Antigen receptors
Antigen-receptor interaction
Recognition of self vs. non-self
The secondary antibody response

Additional Reading

Ashwell, J.D. and Weissman, A.M. 1996. Chapter 5. T cell antigen receptor genes, gene products, and coreceptors. In Rich, R.R. (ed.) Clinical Immunology: Principles and Practice. Mosby-Year Book, St. Louis.

Hay, F. 1996. Chapter 6. The Generation of Diversity. In Roitt, I., Brostoff, J., and Male, D., (eds.) Immunology. 4th ed. Mosby-Year Book, St. Louis.

TERMS:

Allele	Many genes may be present in an individual in one of several sequences. Each sequence possibility is called an allele.
Combinatorial Diversity	Antigen receptor diversity that is created by the combination of different protein chains that make up the antigen receptor complex.
Junctional Diversity	Antigen receptor diversity that is created when segments of DNA that form antigen receptor genes are spliced together at different nucleic acid base pairs.
Somatic Mutation	Alterations in gene sequences such as base pair substitutions, deletions, or additions. Somatic mutation also increases antigen receptor diversity.

Study Questions

1. What is the basic structure of B cell and T cell antigen receptor genes?
2. What processes during the genetic modification of antigen receptor genes contribute to the diversification of antigen receptor specificities?
3. Why does only a very small percentage of lymphocyte precursors mature to possess antigen receptors with unique specificities?

TOPIC 4: Clonal Development of Lymphocytes

Principles

1. B and T lymphocytes divide to produce large clones (approximately 10^9 in mammals).
2. Lymphocytes of the same clone recognize exactly the same antigens.
3. Clonal expansion after exposure to an antigen is a means of increasing the number of lymphocytes that are reactive against that antigen.

4. Increased numbers of cells in the clones that recognize an antigen is the basis for immunological memory.

Explanation

As was discussed in the previous topic, mammals generate lymphocytes with millions of different antigenic specificities. This is necessary so that the immune system will be prepared at all times to recognize and respond to any foreign antigens that may invade the host animal. It is this tremendous diversity, however, that necessarily limits the number of lymphocytes in circulation that are capable of responding to any given antigen. The immune system needs a mechanism whereby it can continually replenish old, dying lymphocytes without risk of losing antigenic specificity and whereby large numbers of lymphocytes reactive against a specific antigen can be produced if the host is exposed to that antigen. Lymphocytes meet these needs by dividing to form identical progeny cells, a process called *cloning*.

It would be inefficient for an animal to produce by random chance from undifferentiated precursors enough lymphocytes with a given antigenic specificity to ward off a large antigenic challenge. Also, lymphocytes are continually lost from circulation and must be replenished. By maintaining clones of diverse lymphocytes, the host always has ready access to the cells that it needs to meet the ever-changing threat of infectious agents.

Under resting conditions, lymphocytes proliferate at a slow, steady rate so that populations of each clone are continually available for surveillance of foreign antigens within the host. When an animal is exposed to a foreign antigen, however, lymphocytes that recognize that antigen are then activated. Activated lymphocytes proliferate at a greater rate than do resting lymphocytes, causing clonal expansion of antigen-specific lymphocytes. The immune system uses the increased numbers of antigen-specific lymphocytes in its attempt to eliminate the foreign antigen from the host.

Clonal expansion of lymphocytes takes place within secondary lymphoid tissues (e.g., lymph nodes). If an infection is localized, the greatest proliferative response will occur within the lymph node(s) receiving drainage from the infected site. Activated lymphocytes proliferate to form dense clusters of cells, called *germinal centers,* within the lymph node. The newly formed antigen-specific lymphocytes may then be released from the lymph node to circulate to the infected site.

After the immune system has eliminated an antigen from the host, lymphocytes are no longer activated, their proliferation rate decreases, and the number of antigen-specific lymphocytes in the host slowly decreases. However, the antigen-specific population does not revert completely to its preexposure state. Certain lymphocytes within the reactive clones are converted to memory lymphocytes and remain within the immune system for long periods.

Memory lymphocytes help the immune system respond more strongly and more quickly when the host animal is exposed again to the same antigen. Memory cells help to form a larger base population of antigen-specific lymphocytes from which to mount an immune response, especially if subsequent antigen exposure occurs shortly after the initial exposure. If the time between antigen exposures is longer, the base population tends to decrease proportionally, but it still will probably be larger than that of a naive (unexposed) animal. Because clonal expansion is exponential, absolute growth within a clone is greater with a larger base population (Fig. 3-5). Memory cells are also more easily activated on exposure to antigen than are naive lymphocytes, so there is less lag time between entry of antigen into the host and the initiation of an immune response against the antigen.

TERM:

Clonal Expansion   Division of cells into identical progeny cells at a rate greater than cells are removed from a population; an increase in the number of cells derived from a common parent cell.

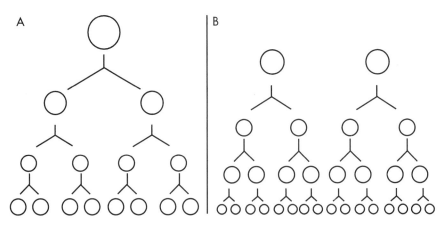

Fig. 3-5   Kinetics of clonal expansion. Given the same number of cell divisions, a larger pool of effector cells can be obtained from a larger base population (group B vs. group A).

Study Questions:

1. Under what conditions and where does clonal expansion of lymphocytes take place?
2. Explain why the immune system responds more rapidly to a second exposure to antigen (immunological memory).
3. Why doesn't the immune system maintain large numbers of cells in all of the clones of lymphocytes so that the individual would have stronger immunity to everything?

TOPIC 5: T Lymphocyte Antigen Recognition

Principles

1. T lymphocytes are capable only of recognizing small pieces of antigen that have been processed and presented by genetically matched antigen-presenting cells.
2. Antigen-presenting cells degrade whole antigens into small fragments that lymphocytes can recognize.
3. Antigen-presenting cells combine antigen fragments with major histocompatibility complex (MHC) molecules for presentation to T lymphocytes.
4. T lymphocytes only recognize antigens that are presented on cells possessing MHC molecules identical to those of the lymphocyte.
5. There is great genetic diversity of MHC molecules among individuals of the same species.

Explanation

Lymphocytes are activated when they bind to their complementary antigens via their antigen receptors (membrane-bound antibody molecules for B lymphocytes and T-cell receptors for T lymphocytes). This binding is very specific and depends on a close structural fit between antigen and receptor molecules. B lymphocytes are capable of binding with antigens in their native conformation. T lymphocytes, however, can only recognize antigens after they have been degraded, processed, and presented on the surface of specialized cells called *antigen-presenting cells (APCs)*.

Several types of cells can function as APCs. Some types, such as dendritic cells and macrophages, are called *professional APCs* and can always present antigen to T lymphocytes. Other cells, such as epithelial cells and B lymphocytes, under resting conditions, do not act as APCs but can be stimulated within sites of inflammation or infection to present antigen to T lymphocytes.

There are two main processing pathways, endogenous and exogenous, by which antigen can be processed by APCs. Each pathway uses its own biochemical degradation processes and unique route of antigen transport through the intracellular organelles of the APC, but both pathways degrade antigenic proteins into fragments (approximately 8 to 20 amino acids in length for the exogenous pathway and 9 to 11 amino acids in length for the endogenous pathway). The antigenic fragments are then combined with host cell molecules, called *major histocompatibility complex (MHC) molecules,* and transported to the surface of the APC where they are bound to the cell membrane.

The endogenous pathway is used to process antigens that have been synthesized within the APC (Fig. 3-6). Viral antigens are included in this category because viruses direct the APCs that they infect to produce viral

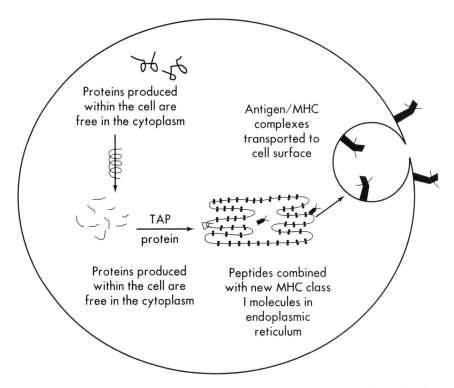

Fig. 3-6   Endogenous pathway of antigen processing. Antigens synthesized within the antigen-presenting cells are processed inside structures called proteosomes. Transporter proteins (TAP) facilitate movement of peptides from the proteosome to the endoplasmic reticulum, where the peptides are combined with MHC class I molecules. The antigen/MHC complexes are then transported to the surface of the antigen-presenting cell.

proteins in addition to the APC's own proteins. The endogenous pathway combines antigenic fragments with class I MHC molecules.

The exogenous pathway is used to process antigens that have been internalized by APCs as preformed molecules (Fig. 3-7). Extracellular bacteria are included in this category because these bacteria replicate outside of the APC and are internalized after their component antigens have been synthesized. The exogenous pathway combines antigens with class II MHC molecules.

The categorization of antigen types and MHC classes with their respective processing pathways is applicable in most instances but is not absolute. Occasionally an endogenously produced antigen is expressed on the surface of an APC with a class II MHC molecule or an exogenous

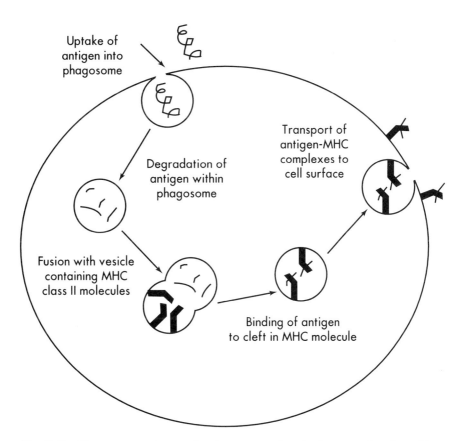

Fig. 3-7 Exogenous pathway of antigen processing. Antigens produced outside of the antigen-presenting cell are internalized, processed, and presented in combination with MHC class II molecules on the surface of the antigen-presenting cell.

protein is expressed with a class I MHC molecule. It is unclear whether these occurrences are the result of an aberration in the major processing pathways or if other, as yet uncharacterized, pathways may be used to process some antigens.

T lymphocytes recognize antigen fragments and MHC molecules on the surface of APCs as combined entities. The antigen fragment lies within a groove of the three-dimensional structure of the MHC molecule. The antigen/MHC complex must fit closely with the antigen-specific portion of the T-cell receptor and its closely associated CD4 or CD8 molecule. CD4 and CD8 molecules bind to MHC molecules, CD4 molecules with class II MHC molecules, and CD8 with class I MHC molecules. Both the antigen specificity and the MHC class must be complementary to the T-cell receptor for lymphocyte activation to occur.

The major histocompatibility molecule expressed on the antigen-presenting cell must match that of the responding T lymphocyte if the lymphocyte is to be activated. Histocompatibility molecules provide a molecular fingerprint to identify cells from a particular host. All cells within an individual have the same collection of histocompatibility markers, but other individuals express a different collection of markers. Histocompatibility molecules are so diverse that practically everyone, except identical twins, has unique markers. There are major and minor histocompatibility molecules; lymphocytes utilize two classes (class I and class II) of MHC molecules in their recognition process.

Genetic restriction of T lymphocyte recognition may have evolved because of the types of functions that T lymphocytes perform. Helper T lymphocytes secrete cytokines, which are molecules that facilitate communication between cells of the immune system. Cytokines may stimulate other cells to proliferate or to be more effective in their ability to destroy foreign antigens. However, cytokines, which are normally secreted in very low concentrations, are active only across relatively short distances, so cells must be close to the T lymphocytes that are releasing cytokines to be affected. Cytotoxic T lymphocytes destroy virally infected cells by a process that also requires close physical contact with target cells. If T lymphocytes must recognize MHC molecules as well as antigen to be activated, this ensures that T cells will only be activated when cells that can be affected by their activation are present.

The differential properties between class I and class II MHC molecules are used to define further the conditions that are appropriate for lymphocyte activation. Class I molecules are expressed by nearly every cell type in the body. Therefore, virally infected cells of nearly any tissue can be recognized and destroyed by cytotoxic T lymphocytes, which usually recognize antigen in combination with class I MHC molecules. Class II MHC molecules, however, are largely restricted to cells of the immune system. Therefore, helper T lymphocytes, which usually recognize antigen in combination with class II MHC molecules, are activated only when other immune cells, which could react to cytokines released by helper T lymphocytes, are present.

Even though one can understand why the association of antigen recognition with MHC molecules is beneficial in localizing T lymphocyte responses to sites where they will be most beneficial, immunologists are not certain why the MHC molecule of the APC must be genetically identical to that of the T lymphocyte. Under physiological conditions, however, antigens would, of necessity, be presented by cells expressing the same MHC molecules because cells with other MHC specificities would not be present within the host. Interestingly, the same T lymphocytes that are MHC-restricted with regard to antigen recognition may also be activated by several MHC molecules that are different from their own in the *absence* of antigen. This phenomenon is known as *alloreactivity* and is discussed in more detail in the topic on transplantation.

Related Topics

Antigen receptors
Antigen-receptor interaction
Helper T lymphocytes
Cytokines
Cytotoxic T lymphocytes
Transplantation

Additional Reading

Germain, R.N. 1994. MHC-dependent antigen processing and peptide presentation: providing ligands for T lymphocyte activation. Cell. 76:287-299.
Golub, E.S. and Green, D.R. 1991. Chapter 20. Antigen processing and presentation. In Immunology: A Synthesis. 2nd ed. Sinauer Associates, Sunderland, Mass.
Monaco, J.J. 1995. Pathways for the processing and presentation of antigens to T cells. J. Leukoc. Biol. 57:543-547.
Rich, R.R. 1996. Chapter 1. The human immune response. In Rich, R.R. (ed.) Clinical Immunology: Principles and Practice. Mosby-Year Book, St. Louis.

TERMS:

Antigen-Presenting Cells (APC)	Cells that process antigens into peptides and express them on their cell surfaces in conjunction with their histocompatibility molecules for presentation to T lymphocytes. T lymphocytes

can recognize antigens only when they are properly presented on APCs.

Antigen Processing	The conversion of antigens into peptides and the combination of the peptides with MHC molecules, creating an antigenic form that is recognizable by T lymphocytes.
Major Histocompatibility Complex (MHC)	Collection of genes that produce proteins involved in antigen recognition by lymphocytes and rejection of grafted tissues.

Study Questions

1. Why are antigen-presenting cells necessary for the activation of T lymphocytes by antigen?
2. How might the replication mode (intracellular vs. extracellular) of an invading infectious organism affect the type of immune response that is generated against it?
3. Why can't antigen-presenting cells from one individual effectively present antigens to a T cell from a genetically different animal?

TOPIC 6: Costimulatory Signals for Lymphocytes

Principles

1. Both B and T lymphocytes must recognize antigen and receive costimulatory signals to produce an immune response.
2. The nature of costimulatory signals influences the type of immune response that is generated.
3. Requirements for costimulation are reduced in previously activated lymphocytes.
4. Helper T lymphocytes that recognize antigen are an important source of costimulatory signals for B lymphocytes.

Explanation

Resting lymphocytes must receive two types of stimulatory signals before they can be fully activated to generate a functional immune response. One signal is provided via the antigen receptor when a lymphocyte binds to its complementary antigen. This signal provides antigen specificity to the activation process. The second signal, called the *costimulatory signal*, is transmitted through cell surface molecules distinct from the antigen receptor and is not antigen specific. Activation of lymphocytes may be further influenced by the presence of various cytokines in the environment of the lymphocyte.

Costimulatory molecules are best characterized for T lymphocytes. Two cell-surface molecules of T lymphocytes, CD28 and CTLA4, have been shown to transmit costimulatory signals when they bind to their complementary molecules (ligands). Several other, as yet undefined, molecules also may participate in the transmission of T cell costimulatory signals. CD28 and CTLA4 have at least two possible ligands, and both ligands are molecules belonging to the B7 family.

B7 molecules are expressed on the surfaces of antigen-presenting cells. Dendritic cells that reside within lymphoid tissues, which are very powerful antigen-presenting cells, express B7 molecules constitutively. Other antigen-presenting cells, such as macrophages, B lymphocytes, and dendritic cells in nonlymphoid tissues can be induced to express B7 molecules on activation. Two different types of B7 molecules have been identified to date: CD80 and CD86.

Both the antigen-specific signal and the costimulatory signal must be received to activate a resting lymphocyte (Fig. 3-8). Stimulation through the antigen receptor in the absence of costimulation causes the lympho-cyte to become anergic (inactivated) or to die. Likewise, delivery of costimulatory signals without antigen-specific binding will not induce lymphocyte activation. Stimulatory signals are most potent when the antigen and the costimulatory molecule to which the lymphocyte binds are located on the same cell.

Once a T lymphocyte has been activated, it can perform its effector function (cytotoxicity or cytokine secretion) on subsequent contact with its complementary antigen even if the cell on which the antigen is located cannot deliver costimulation. The initial two-signal requirement prob-ably helps to prevent inappropriate activation of the immune system, but once activated, T lymphocytes must be able to direct their immune defenses against any type of infected or abnormal cell and not just those bearing costimulatory molecules.

B lymphocytes also require a type of costimulation, but this is usually provided by helper T lymphocytes. B cell responses to most antigens (T-dependent antigens) require T cell help to induce significant antibody production. This help is provided through secreted cytokines and direct cellular contact between B and T cells. B lymphocytes require stimulation through binding a molecule called CD40, but this is usually provided through contact with helper T cells.

Many microbial substances are potent stimulators of costimulatory activity, which enhances the ability of the immune system to react to their presence in the host. Lipopolysaccharide, which is a component of the

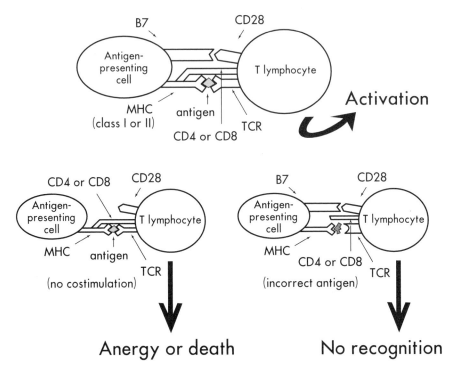

Fig. 3-8   Lymphocytes must receive an antigen-specific signal through their antigen receptor (TCR) and a nonspecific costimulatory signal to be activated.

cell walls of gram-negative bacteria, induces B7 expression on certain antigen-presenting cells. However, other microorganisms may downregulate costimulatory activity as a means of evading immune attack. For example, certain *Leishmania* sp. inhibit costimulatory molecule expression on macrophages. This would render affected macrophages presenting leishmanial antigens to lymphocytes less likely to activate antigen-specific lymphocytes and more likely to induce anergy in these cells.

The two-signal model is probably an oversimplification of the activation process. Because there are multiple types of costimulatory molecules on lymphocytes and multiple types of ligands on antigen-presenting cells, it is probable that there are qualitative differences in the signals that are generated through each molecule. Little is known about the biochemical events that occur after binding between costimulatory receptors and their ligands, but it is evident that costimulatory signals are an important regulatory control on the activation process. For example, CTLA-4 has been identified as a costimulatory receptor capable of activating naive T lymphocytes. However, binding of CTLA-4 to B7 ligands late in the immune response can inhibit further T cell activation, which provides a negative feedback mechanism to control the magnitude of an immune response.

Lymphocyte responses to antigen binding and costimulation also depend on the state of differentiation of the lymphocyte and the types of cytokines present in the local environment at the time of activation. Lymphocytes may react in different ways to the same environmental stimuli at different points during their maturation process. They may also follow different maturation pathways depending on the types of cytokines to which they are exposed during the activation process (e.g., Th1 vs. Th2 cells). Thus the cumulative effect of maturation state, cellular signaling, and input from soluble cytokines not only determines whether the lymphocyte is activated or rendered anergic but also influences what function(s) the activated cell will perform.

It is still unclear how cellular signaling and soluble cytokines work together to mold an immune response, and it is undoubtedly a complex and dynamic event. However, immunologists continue to seek understanding of the activation process because manipulation of lymphocyte activation could lead to new strategies to treat inappropriate immune responses (e.g., hypersensitivities and autoimmunity) and new approaches for vaccine design.

Related Topics

Antigen receptors
T lymphocyte antigen recognition
Helper T lymphocyte subsets

Additional Reading

Janeway, C.A. Jr. and Bottomly, K. 1994. Signals and signs for lymphocyte responses. Cell. 76:275-285.
Kaye, P.M. 1995. Costimulation and the regulation of antimicrobial immunity. Immunol. Today. 16:423-427.
Nickoloff, B.J. and Turka, L.A. 1994. Immunological functions of non-professional antigen-presenting cells: new insights from studies of T-cell interactions with keratinocytes. Immunol. Today. 15:464-469.

TERM:

Costimulation	Second stimulatory signal, which is not antigen-specific, that must be received by lymphocytes in addition to antigen-specific stimulation for proper activation.

Study Questions

1. How do the requirements for costimulatory signals differ between a primary and secondary immune response?
2. What is a major source of costimulatory signals for a T lymphocyte?
3. What is a major source of costimulatory signals for a B lymphocyte?
4. What happens if a naive lymphocyte recognizes an antigen in the absence of costimulatory signals?
5. Why would multiple receptors and ligands for costimulation be advantageous for the immune system?

TOPIC 7: Superantigens

Principles

1. Superantigens from bacteria and viruses are antigens that activate multiple clones of T lymphocytes.
2. Superantigens are not recognized by T lymphocytes in the same manner as conventional antigens.
3. Large-scale immune activation by superantigens can cause severe clinical disease.
4. Superantigens cross-link MHC and T-cell receptor molecules by binding to each of them outside of the normal antigen-binding site.

Explanation

Superantigen is the collective term used to characterize a diverse group of antigens that can activate large proportions of T lymphocytes within an individual. Whereas any given conventional antigen activates less than 1% of the total lymphocyte pool, superantigens activate 5% to 20% of all lymphocytes. Antigens that induce powerful proliferative responses in lymphocytes were described as early as 1969, but it wasn't until the late 1980s that the significance of these responses was appreciated and the term superantigen was adopted. Intense research into the stimulatory mechanisms of these antigens and their potential roles in disease processes continues today.

T lymphocytes do not recognize superantigens in the same manner that they recognize conventional antigens. The antigen receptor (TCR) of most T lymphocytes is composed of alpha and beta protein chains, and these chains are highly diverse. The antigen-binding site for conventional antigens is dependent on the three-dimensional structure of the combined chains and usually involves amino acids located on each chain. Thus, conventional antigen-binding sites can assume millions of different conformations and antigen specificities, and very few lymphocytes are specific for any particular antigen. Superantigens, however, do not bind to the conventional antigen-binding site of the TCR (Fig. 3-9). They bind only to a specific segment (V segment) of the beta chain, and different superantigens preferentially bind to different V_β segments. Because of this, the diversity of superantigen-binding sites is necessarily more restricted than their conventional counterparts. Only a limited number of genes code for V_β, and, unlike conventional antigens, superantigen specificity of a TCR is not significantly affected by the combination of specific V_β segments with other beta segments or with various alpha chains. (Lymphocytes stimulated by a given superantigen may preferentially express certain alpha chains, but the significance of this finding is unknown.) Therefore, there are many more lymphocytes within a

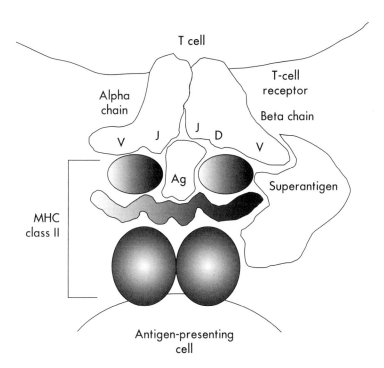

Fig. 3-9   A cross-sectional view of the interactions between conventional peptide antigen, TCR, and MHC. Peptide sits within a groove in the MHC molecule. Superantigens are not processed to peptides and therefore are not presented in the antigen groove. Instead, they bind to more conserved sites on the side of the MHC class II molecule and interact primarily with the V_β region of the TCR. (From Rich, R.R. [ed.] 1996. Clinical Immunology: Principles and Practice. Mosby-Year Book, St. Louis.)

population that have the proper V_β segment necessary to recognize a specific superantigen than there are lymphocytes with the overall TCR structure necessary to recognize a given conventional antigen. A similar binding mechanism is probably used with gamma/delta lymphocytes that are reactive against superantigens.

Superantigens must be presented bound to class II MHC molecules on the surface of antigen-presenting cells to activate T lymphocytes, but superantigens bind to class II MHC molecules outside of the groove used to bind conventional antigens. At least two distinct binding sites have been characterized; superantigens may use one or the other or bind to both with different strengths (affinities). The sites on the MHC molecule to which superantigens bind contain highly conserved amino acid sequences and conformation because superantigens can be successfully presented to T lymphocytes by antigen-presenting cells from different individuals or even from different animal species. The process does not appear to be entirely unrestricted though, because certain allelic forms of MHC molecules bind more strongly to superantigens than others can.

It is believed that superantigens must bind to class II MHC molecules before they can activate T lymphocytes because binding to the MHC molecule alters the conformation of the superantigen so that it can bind correctly to the TCR. Rare instances in which superantigens successfully stimulated T lymphocytes in the absence of MHC molecules have been documented, but it is possible that the superantigen in these reports had been slightly denatured by some other mechanism, thus exposing TCR-binding sites on the antigen.

Presentation in combination with class II MHC molecules restricts the type of cell that can be used as an antigen-presenting cell because class II MHC expression is largely restricted to cells of the immune system. However, superantigens can be successfully presented to lymphocytes that would require presentation of conventional antigens in the context of class I MHC molecules, such as CD8+ T cells. CD8+ lymphocytes can interact with conventional antigen and class II MHC molecules, but the interaction with conventional antigens/class II MHC complexes is so weak that it is physiologically insignificant. However, superantigens bind to T cells with much greater strength than do conventional antigens, so the interaction with CD8+ cells, despite presentation by the "wrong" MHC molecules, is stable enough to elicit a T cell response.

Superantigens differ from conventional antigens in that they are presented to T lymphocytes as intact proteins. They do not require processing into peptide fragments within the antigen-presenting cell before they can activate T cells.

When superantigens bind successfully to T lymphocytes, they initially induce proliferation and cytokine secretion by these cells. Because so many lymphocytes are affected by any given superantigen, there is a massive release of cytokines, many of which are proinflammatory, into host tissues. This can cause generalized shock, and even death, in the host. An example of this is the toxic shock syndrome caused by an exotoxin of *Staphylococcus aureus*, a potent superantigen.

After the initial proliferation and cytokine release, affected lymphocytes become "exhausted" and refractory to further stimulation. This nonresponsive state is called *anergy*. Sometimes superantigen-induced anergy is not complete, but it takes stimuli that are ten- to 100-fold stronger than the initial stimulus to induce an immune response by these cells. Because lymphocytes that are responsive to many different conventional antigens may become anergic after exposure to a single superantigen, the host may appear clinically immunodeficient to many different infectious agents after a severe immune response against a superantigen.

The ability of superantigens to induce anergic states in affected lymphocytes has been used as a model to study immune tolerance. It has been hypothesized that superantigen-like activity occurs when the developing fetus discriminates between self and non-self antigens. Self antigens in the developing thymus act like superantigens, causing lymphocytes that recognize that antigen to become anergic or die. A similar mechanism may occur outside of the thymus so that lymphocytes reactive against self antigens that are continually present in the host are deleted and lost from the T cell repertoire.

Superantigens of bacterial and viral origin have been characterized, and several other antigens have been considered as potential superantigens. The best characterized superantigens are certain toxins produced by *Staphylococcus aureus* and *Streptococcus pyogenes*. Superantigens produced by *Mycoplasma arthritidis, Pseudomonas aeruginosa,* and *Clostridium perfringens* have also been proposed. The best described viral superantigen is produced by a murine retrovirus, the mouse mammary tumor virus; the nucleoprotein (G protein) of the rabies virus has also been implicated. It is probable that there are many other infectious agents that also produce superantigens. The known superantigens are very different structurally, which is somewhat unusual for sets of molecules that have similar functions.

There are several reasons why it would be beneficial for an infectious agent to produce a superantigen. If the host undergoes widespread, generalized lymphocyte activation early after infection, it may be disabled from mounting a coordinated immune response that is directed specifically against the inciting infectious agent. After the affected lymphocytes become anergic, the host may be rendered immunodeficient, which would enhance the chance for survival of the pathogen within the host.

Superantigens may increase the number of host cells that a virus can infect. Certain viruses, including the human immunodeficiency virus (HIV) and related immunodeficiency viruses of domestic animals, preferentially infect lymphocytes. If the viruses induce widespread lymphocyte proliferation early in infection, the number of available host cells increases. It has been proposed that the g120 protein of HIV may act as a superantigen. If this hypothesis is verified, it may lead to a new avenue of research for possible preventive and therapeutic treatment strategies against AIDS.

Superantigens have also been implicated as causative factors in autoimmune diseases. Stimulation by superantigens may activate a heretofore dormant self-reactive lymphocyte population or may stimulate the proliferation of lymphocytes that are cross-reactive with self antigens. However, direct evidence for such roles is still scant.

Nearly all of our knowledge about superantigens involves interactions with T lymphocytes. It is probable that superantigens that stimulate B lymphocytes also exist, but this possibility is largely conceptual at this time. As more is learned about superantigens and their ability to manipulate the immune system, immunologists may be able to use superantigen-like molecules to augment weak immune responses or to control undesirable immune responses in a regulated manner.

Related Topics

Antigen receptors
Antigen receptor diversity

Additional Reading

Fleischer, B. 1994. Superantigens. APMIS. 102:3-12.

Goodglick, L. and Braun, J. 1994. Revenge of the microbes: superantigens of the T and B cell lineage. Am. J. Pathol. 144(4):623-636.

Scherer, M.T., Ignatowicz, L., and Winslow, G.M. 1993. Superantigens: bacterial and viral proteins that manipulate the immune system. Annu. Rev. Cell Biol. 9:101-128.

Uchiyama, T., Yan, X.J., Imanishi, K., and Yagi, J. 1994. Bacterial superantigens: mechanism of T cell activation by the superantigens and their role in the pathogenesis of infectious diseases. Microbiol. Immunol. 38:245-256.

Webb, S.R. and Gascoigne, N.R.J. 1994. T-cell activation by superantigens. Curr. Opin. Immunol. 6:467-475.

TERM:

Superantigen	A special type of antigen that binds to lymphocytes outside of the traditional binding site and that stimulates large populations of lymphocytes.

Study Questions

1. How does binding of superantigens to lymphocytes differ from that of conventional antigens?
2. How might possession of a superantigen be advantageous for pathogenic organisms?
3. What are some of the consequences of superantigen-induced activation of T lymphocytes?

TOPIC 8: Recognition of Self vs. Non-Self

Principles

1. The immune system does not normally react to self antigens. This is known as tolerance.
2. The immune system learns to distinguish self from non-self primarily during fetal development.
3. The process of thymic selection eliminates T lymphocytes that recognize self.
4. Non-self antigens residing within an individual before T and B lymphocytes mature during fetal development are treated as self antigens by the developing immune system.

Explanation

The immune system is a powerful weapon against infectious agents and neoplastic (cancerous) cells. It constantly monitors the body for abnormal (foreign) antigens and attempts to destroy them so that the body maintains homeostasis. Because it is such a powerful weapon, the immune system must be carefully directed. The same forces that are beneficial in eliminating foreign antigens could be very detrimental if they were directed against the normal tissues of the host. Therefore, the developing immune system of the fetus must learn to discriminate between normal fetal tissues (self antigens) and foreign, or non-self, antigens and must keep lymphocytes that are reactive against self antigens from destroying the fetus.

Antigen receptor specificities are generated randomly within developing lymphocytes. Consequently, lymphocytes reactive against practically any antigen, whether it is foreign or a normal constituent of the individual, may be produced. However, T lymphocytes undergo a selection process within the thymus as they develop, wherein lymphocytes possessing useless or harmful antigen receptors are destroyed while those expressing receptors specific for antigens not present in the fetus are allowed to mature.

Thymic selection begins early in lymphocyte development. After antigen receptor genes undergo random genetic rearrangement, only those lymphocytes with functional rearrangements are allowed to proceed to the next step in development. This selection step, although not antigen specific, prevents the production of lymphocytes bearing nonfunctional antigen receptors or no antigen receptors at all.

Once lymphocytes have reached the stage in development in which they bear functional antigen receptors on their cell surfaces, antigen-specific selection begins. Thymic selection includes positive and negative selection components (Fig. 3-10). During positive selection, lymphocytes reactive against antigens presented with self MHC molecules are stimulated to mature and/or be rescued from programmed cell death (apoptosis). In the negative selection phase, lymphocytes reactive against self antigens are eliminated. Usually self-reactive lymphocytes are eliminated by programmed cell death, but some self-reactive lymphocytes undergo functional inactivation instead.

Lymphocytes are selected either for death or maturation when their antigen receptors bind with complexes of antigenic peptides and major histocompatibility complex (MHC) molecules on antigen-presenting cells within the thymus. Recognition of self MHC molecules is required for both positive and negative selection. As one would expect, if lymphocytes recognize self MHC molecules bound to the appropriate self peptides, they are eliminated. One might envision that positive selection occurs after interactions with self MHC in the absence of self peptides. However, the signaling mechanisms for thymic selection are far more complex than that, and as yet unclear. The affinity, or strength, with which lymphocytes bind to antigen/MHC complexes may affect selection processes, as may the density of antigen receptors on the lymphocyte, the type of peptide that forms a complex with the MHC molecule, or the duration of contact between the lymphocyte and antigen/MHC complex. Small quantitative differences in these factors could also substantially affect the selection process.

Certain types of cells within the thymus that act as antigen-presenting cells for developing lymphocytes may influence positive or negative selection. Cortical epithelial cells are potent inducers of positive

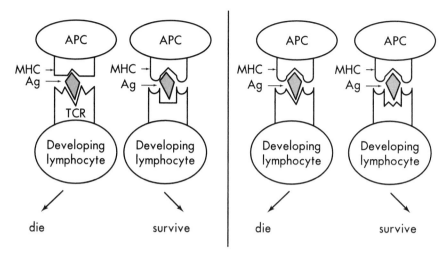

Fig. 3-10 Two-stage selection of developing lymphocytes based on binding characteristics of the TCR. **A,** Positive selection. Lymphocytes with TCRs capable of binding to some specific self MHC molecule (class I or class II) expressed by the antigen-presenting cell (cortical epithelial cell) are positively selected; all other developing lymphocytes are eliminated. The antigen in this figure is a self antigen. **B,** Negative selection. Developing lymphocytes that display TCRs that can bind to self MHC molecules plus some self antigen are negatively selected (i.e., die). The antigen-presenting cell for negative selection is often a thymic hematopoietic cell. Those few lymphocytes that survive both positive and negative selection are released to secondary lymphoid tissues. (Modified from Rich, R.R. [ed.] 1996. Clinical Immunology: Principles and Practice. Mosby-Year Book, St. Louis.)

selection; thymic cells of hematopoietic (bone marrow) origin are more likely to induce negative selection. These distinctions are not absolute, because several antigen-presenting cell types can mediate positive and negative selection, but cortical epithelium and thymic hematopoietic cells appear most likely to mediate positive and negative selection, respectively, in vivo.

Closely associated with positive selection is the process whereby lymphocytes are committed to express either CD4 or CD8 receptors. Immature lymphocytes go through a developmental stage in which they express CD4 and CD8 receptors simultaneously. As they mature, they lose their ability to express one receptor or the other. Expression of CD4 or CD8 is closely, although not absolutely, associated with the final effector function of the lymphocyte. The selection process whereby a lymphocyte is committed to express CD4 or CD8 is also highly uncertain. It is possible that different developmental pathways are required for maturation into each type of cell.

Immunologists previously thought that selection occurred only in the T lymphocyte lineage. They thought that the reactivity of B lymphocytes was controlled indirectly, through the actions of helper T lymphocytes. Self-reactive B lymphocytes would not be induced to produce significant quantities of autoantibodies if the appropriate antigen-specific T lymphocytes were not available to provide stimulatory cytokines or cell-cell contacts. Although it is true that helper T lymphocytes do influence proliferation and final maturation of most B lymphocytes, it is also apparent that a type of lymphocyte selection also occurs within the bone marrow. This process is even less understood than thymic selection, but it is believed to include components similar to thymic selection.

Discrimination between self and non-self antigens occurs during fetal life. It is typically during the second trimester that the fetal immune system becomes mature enough to discriminate self from non-self and to initiate lymphocyte selection processes. During the period of antigenic discrimination, all antigens currently residing within the fetus are considered to be self antigens. For the most part, this is an accurate assumption because the fetus lives in a highly protected local environment and should be relatively sheltered from entry by foreign antigens. However, the period of antigenic discrimination is also a time when the immune system can be fooled into accepting foreign antigens as normal constituents of the host. If a fetus is infected with a microbial agent or has genetically foreign cells in its circulation at that time, the immune system will consider these antigens, along with the normal host antigens of the individual, to be self antigens. Lymphocytes reactive against these antigens will be eliminated, and the immune system will never mount an immune response against them.

Several clinical examples demonstrate the ability of the fetus to accept, or become tolerant of, foreign antigens in utero. A classical example is that of fraternal twin calves that become tolerant of each other's antigens. Fraternal twin calves share common placental vasculature. Therefore, genetically distinct blood cells from each calf are mixed in fetal circulation. If these calves were the product of separate gestations, each would be immunologically distinct and would recognize the unique antigens of the other calf as foreign. However, because each calf was exposed to blood cells of the other during the time of immune discrimination, they recognize all of each other's antigens as their own. They behave immunologically as if they were identical twins, as evidenced by the fact that each calf will tolerate skin grafts from the other.

Recently, immunologists have begun to question whether discrimination between self and non-self is limited to the fetal period. They have shown that by carefully controlling the antigenic dose and the types of antigen-presenting cells that are present, adult mice can be induced to accept foreign antigens as self. These findings have great implications for the future of immunotherapy against autoimmune disease or transplant rejection because they suggest controlled tolerance to specific antigens is achievable even in adult animals and may be used therapeutically in lieu of generalized immunosuppression.

Some researchers also contend that the concept of immune discrimination of self from non-self should be broadened: the distinguishing criterion may be whether the immune system senses an antigen to be dangerous or not. Under this model, self antigens are tolerated because they are not dangerous whereas foreign antigens induce danger signals that, in turn, induce immune responsiveness to that antigen. The exact nature of the danger signals has yet to be elucidated.

Related Topics

Antigen receptor diversity
Autoimmunity
Transplantation

Additional Reading

Pennisi, E. 1996. Teetering on the brink of danger. Science. 271:1665-1667.
Robey, E. and Fowlkes, B.J. 1994. Selective events in T cell development. Annu. Rev. Immunol. 12:675-705.
Schwartz, R.H. 1989. Acquisition of immunologic self-tolerance. Cell. 57:1073-1081.

TERMS:

Apoptosis	Programmed cell death.
Thymic Selection	The process whereby immature lymphocytes in the thymus are deleted if they are specific for self antigens or allowed to mature if they recognize foreign antigens.

Study Questions

1. What is the purpose of thymic selection?
2. What is positive selection for T lymphocytes in the thymus?
3. What is negative selection for T lymphocytes in the thymus?

4. Some calves are born with large amounts of bovine viral diarrhea virus in their blood, yet they do not have antibodies to the virus. Why might this occur?

TOPIC 9: Tolerance

Principles

1. An individual's immune system may become tolerant of specific antigens. Tolerance may be temporary or long-lived.
2. Tolerance may be induced centrally (within primary lymphoid tissues during lymphocyte development) or at peripheral sites.
3. Antigens residing in immune-privileged sites are relatively protected from immune attack even though the immune system may attack the same antigens if located elsewhere in the body.
4. Lack of immune response through tolerance is a distinct phenomenon from lack of response caused by immunodeficiency.

Explanation

Because of the random nature of how the specificity of a lymphocyte's antigen receptors are generated, lymphocytes that recognize any given antigen theoretically may be produced within an individual. This is an essential feature of the immune system because it allows an individual to be immunologically prepared to react against any foreign antigen it may encounter. However, it is not desirable to mount an immune response against one's own tissue antigens (self or auto antigens), so the immune system has mechanisms to become tolerant, or nonresponsive, against such antigens.

Immune tolerance can occur in several ways. Autoreactive lymphocytes can be physically eliminated from the individual or they can be functionally inactivated. Tolerance can be induced within the thymus or bone marrow, where lymphocytes develop and mature (central tolerance), or it can be induced in mature lymphocytes that are located throughout the body (peripheral tolerance).

Within the thymus, developing lymphocytes undergo thymic selection, a process in which autoreactive lymphocytes are removed and lymphocytes reacting against foreign antigens are allowed to mature. Thymic selection is the primary mechanism by which immune tolerance of T lymphocytes is achieved. Physical destruction of lymphocytes, also called *clonal deletion,* appears to be the chief method of removing autoreactive lymphocytes from the thymus, although functionally inactive, or anergic, autoreactive cells also have been detected within the thymus. Once a lymphocyte has been marked for destruction, it undergoes a programmed cell death, called *apoptosis,* characterized by fragmentation and dissolution of the cell nucleus. Selection against autoreactive B lymphocytes within the bone marrow (in mammals) or the bursa of Fabricius (in birds) also occurs.

Although centrally induced tolerance is a powerful mechanism for controlling the release of autoreactive lymphocytes, it cannot prevent all autoreactive lymphocytes from reaching peripheral sites. An occasional autoreactive cell escapes detection and removal within primary lymphoid organs. Also, selection against self antigens in the thymus and bone marrow is based on recognition of those antigens that are expressed within those tissues. Other antigens, specific for other tissues of the body, may not be expressed within the thymus or bone marrow, and consequently would not be considered as targets for central tolerance. Therefore, the immune system also has mechanisms to tolerize autoreactive cells within the periphery.

Peripheral tolerance probably occurs most often by functional inactivation, although there is evidence that peripheral clonal deletion does occur. A lymphocyte may become anergic instead of being activated if it encounters its antigen in the absence of activating costimulatory signals. Activating costimulatory signals are supplied by professional antigen-presenting cells, such as macrophages or dendritic cells, which act as scavengers for foreign antigens. However, it is likely that lymphocytes encounter tissue-specific self antigens on the surfaces of parenchymal cells (cells that form the substance of an organ), which may not be able to provide costimulation.

Functional inactivation, whether by anergy or active suppression, may be partial or complete. For example, an anergic lymphocyte may be unable to produce the cytokine interleukin-2 for its own development and maturation, but it may be able to respond to interleukin-2 that is supplied by other sources. Also, the nonresponsiveness of anergic or suppressed lymphocytes may be relative; if an antigenic stimulus is sufficiently potent, or accompanied by the proper costimulatory signals, an immune response still may occur.

Functional inactivation may be temporary or long-lived. Suppression, which is an active process, only lasts as long as the suppressive influences (cells or soluble factors) are present in the environment of the cell. However, anergy may also be temporary. Whereas some anergic cells die off over time, others may eventually regain their functionality. Maintenance of tolerance often depends on continued presence of the tolerizing antigen.

In addition to tolerance to self antigens, which is necessary for an individual's health, the immune system may also become tolerant of certain foreign antigens. The exact mechanisms by which a given foreign antigen induces tolerance, rather than immune responsiveness, within an individual are currently unknown. However, the ease with which a lymphocyte may be tolerized depends on the developmental stage of the lymphocyte, the type and dose of antigen, and the route of antigen administration. Young, developing lymphocytes are more susceptible to tolerizing influences than are mature cells. Soluble antigens are more tolerizing than are particulate antigens, and antigens administered orally or intravenously are more tolerizing than are those administered subcutaneously or intramuscularly. Tolerance tends to occur when antigens are administered in very small or very large doses (called *low-* and *high-dose tolerance,* respectively).

A special type of tolerance to foreign antigens that commonly occurs is called *oral tolerance.* Antigens that are ingested do not tend to induce a systemic immune response after they are absorbed through the intestinal wall, although they may elicit a mild local antibody response, especially IgA, within the intestine. This apparent dichotomy—local responsiveness in the face of systemic nonresponsiveness—may prevent the immune system from overreacting to the myriad dietary antigens that an individual encounters each day while allowing localized immune responses to monitor antigens at the gut surface. A similar phenomenon occurs in response to inhaled antigens. Oral tolerance probably occurs through a combination of active suppression and anergy and is mediated through the actions of T lymphocytes, but the exact mechanism still is unclear.

There are certain sites within the body, called *immune-privileged sites,* where foreign antigens are relatively protected from attack and removal by the immune system. Such sites include the central nervous system, the anterior chamber of the eye, the maternal/fetal interface of the placenta and uterine wall, and the testis. Immune privilege may have evolved as a protective mechanism in sites where inflammation would cause severe impairment to the function of the organ.

Immunologists originally thought that privileged sites were physically sequestered from the cells of the immune system, thus accounting for the ability of foreign tissue grafts and other antigens to survive in these tissues but not in others within the same individual. This theory was supported by the fact that privileged sites are typically characterized by poor or aberrant lymphatic drainage and a blood/tissue barrier that inhibits migration of immune cells into and out of the privileged tissue. However, it is now apparent that no site is completely devoid of immune surveillance, so it is more likely that privileged sites exist because they do not provide the proper environment for immune responses to occur. Cells within privileged sites often have poor or atypical expression of major histocompatibility molecules, so they may not be recognized efficiently by T lymphocytes. Privileged sites are also often characterized by a suppressive microenvironment that inhibits immune responses by cells residing within the environment. Immunologists are still trying to characterize the specific factors responsible for the suppressive environment. Immune tolerance within privileged sites is relative. Certain foreign antigens may exist indefinitely without consequence within privileged sites, but others, particularly those that are highly immunogenic, may last only slightly longer in privileged sites than they would in nonprivileged sites.

Immune tolerance is a powerful mechanism for controlling the reactivity of the immune system. The lack of immune responsiveness induced by immune tolerance, however, is not the same as the nonresponsiveness that occurs in immunodeficiency states. Immune tolerance is an antigen-specific phenomenon, and it is actively controlled. It allows specific immune responses to be depressed while allowing the rest of the immune system to function normally.

Related Topics

Antigen receptor diversity
Costimulatory signals for lymphocytes
Recognition of self vs. non-self
Cytokines

Additional Reading

Goodnow, C.C. 1996. Balancing immunity and tolerance: deleting and tuning lymphocyte repertoires. Proc. Natl. Acad. Sci. U. S. A. 93:2264-2271.
Miller, J.F.A.P. 1992. Peripheral cell tolerance. Annu. Rev. Immunol. 10:51-69.
Steilein, J.W. 1993. Immune privilege as the result of local tissue barriers and immunosuppressive microenvironments. Curr. Opin. Immunol. 5:428-432.
Vacchio, M.S. and Ashwell, J.D. 1994. T cell tolerance. Chem. Immunol. 58:1-33.

TERMS:

Anergy   State of functional inactivation.

Autoreactive   Recognizing self antigens.

Central Tolerance	Nonresponsiveness to a defined antigen that is acquired within primary lymphoid tissues during lymphocyte development. Central tolerance is usually achieved by deleting self-reactive lymphocytes from the lymphocyte pool.
Immune-privileged Site	Specific sites in the body, such as the brain, anterior chamber of the eye, and testis, where antigens are relatively protected from surveillance by the immune system.
Oral Tolerance	Phenomenon in which ingested antigens induce systemic nonresponsiveness, although a mild localized IgA response may occur. Oral tolerance probably evolved as a protective mechanism to prevent an individual from mounting improper immune responses to dietary antigens.
Peripheral Tolerance	Nonresponsiveness to a defined antigen that is acquired outside of the primary lymphoid tissues. Peripheral tolerance is usually achieved by making self-reactive lymphocytes nonfunctional (anergic), even though they physically remain in the lymphocyte population.

Study Questions

1. How does immune tolerance differ from immunodeficiency?
2. What is the difference between centrally and peripherally induced tolerance?
3. What factors influence whether tolerance to a particular antigen will be established?
4. What are immune-privileged sites? Give some examples.
5. What happens if tolerance breaks down and lymphocytes start to react against self antigens?

CHAPTER 4

Effector Mechanisms

In contrast to the fairly uniform function of B lymphocytes (the production of antibodies), T lymphocytes perform widely varying functions. Some T cells kill infected cells directly; others contribute to overall immunity by secreting stimulatory molecules and providing cellular contacts that coordinate activities among the many cells involved in immune responses. Still others down-regulate immune responses to prevent attacks against self antigens and to resolve inflammation once a foreign antigen has been eliminated. Because T lymphocytes are so heterogeneous and many principles governing their actions do not necessarily apply to all T cells equally, immunologists have developed a nomenclature system to define subsets of T lymphocytes. This is somewhat confusing because T lymphocyte subsets are sometimes defined based on cell surface molecules and sometimes based on function. It is becoming apparent that there is some overlap in function between the subsets. Nonetheless, based on function, T lymphocytes are divided into three broad classes: helper (T_h) cells, cytotoxic (T_c) cells, and suppressor (T_s) cells.

Originally, immunologists believed that T lymphocytes performing a certain function could be differentiated from other T lymphocytes by the type of receptor molecules that they express on their surface membranes. They thought that helper T lymphocytes expressed CD4 molecules and recognized antigen bound to class II major histocompatibility complex (MHC) molecules, while cytotoxic and suppressor cells expressed CD8 and recognized MHC class I-bound antigens. Although these rules are useful generalizations and are largely accurate, we now know that some CD8+ T cells perform helper functions, and occasionally CD4+ cells participate in certain types of cytotoxicity. Probably the most heterogeneous in phenotype though are the supressor T lymphocytes. Some texts refrain from using the term *suppressor cell* because it is now evident that immune suppression is not the function of a single cell. Rather, suppression is a broad, multifaceted aspect of immune regulation that can be effected by many types of lymphocytes, as well as other cells, depending on the local environment around those cells.

In this collection of topics, we will discuss the various functions of classical T lymphocytes. We will also discuss gamma/delta lymphocytes, which have an alternative form of T-cell receptor and for which functions are yet largely undefined, and intraepithelial lymphocytes, which recently have garnered attention for their functional niche because of the anatomical location at which they effect their immunological responses.

List of Principles

Classes of Antibody

B lymphocytes respond to antigen by producing antibodies. There are five major classes of antibodies, each with different roles in host defense.

Antibodies protect individuals from disease by inactivating infectious organisms or by helping other components of the immune system to eliminate organisms from the body.

Helper T Lymphocytes

Helper T lymphocytes respond to antigens by secreting many different cytokines in different combinations and participating in cell-cell contacts that orchestrate cell-mediated immunity.

Helper T lymphocytes enable B lymphocytes to produce strong antibody responses to most antigens.

Signals from helper T lymphocytes make other leukocytes more aggressive and efficient.

Cytokines

Cytokines are small, soluble molecules that provide a means of molecular communication between cells. There are many families of cytokine molecules.

An individual cytokine may be produced by several cell types.

Cytokines have multiple and overlapping functions. Cytokines may even induce the production of other cytokines.

Cytokines affect those cells that have specific receptor molecules for them.

List of Principles — cont'd

Cytokines in low concentration will produce a local effect and in higher concentration may produce a systemic effect.

Helper T Lymphocyte Subsets

Helper T lymphocytes may be divided into T_h1 and T_h2 subsets based on whether they primarily induce a cell-mediated immune response or an antibody response.

Each subset secretes a distinct combination of cytokines. In the continuum between pure T_h1 and pure T_h2 responses, most immune responses are characterized by a mixture of the two responses.

Cytotoxic T Lymphocytes

Cytotoxic T lymphocytes respond to foreign antigens presented on cell surfaces by killing the cells that produced the antigens.

Cytotoxic T lymphocytes differ from natural killer cells in that they kill cells in an antigen-specific manner.

At least two mechanisms are used by cytotoxic T lymphocytes to kill target cells (the perforin-mediated pathway and the FAS-mediated pathway).

Natural Killer (NK) Cells

Natural killer cells are a component of the native defense mechanisms that help to control virus-infected and cancer cells without previous exposure to the antigens on these cells. Natural killer cells cannot recognize and attack free viruses or other microorganisms.

Natural killer cells are a subset of lymphocytes, but unlike B and T lymphocytes, they do not recognize specific foreign antigenic epitopes and they do not undergo clonal expansion after the first exposure to antigen.

Antigen recognition by NK cells is not thoroughly understood, but they seem to kill cells that fail to adequately express normal self antigens on their surface.

NK cells look like large granular lymphocytes and use the contents of their granules to kill target cells by inserting pores in target membranes and by inducing apoptosis (programmed cell death) in target cells.

NK cell activity is increased in the presence of specific antibody against cell surface antigens and by interferon and some other cytokines.

Continued

▬ List of Principles — cont'd ▬

Gamma/Delta Gamma/delta T lymphocytes may recognize antigen in a
T Lymphocytes manner different from alpha/beta T lymphocytes.

Immunologists have speculated that, because of their affinity for epithelial locations and their unique TCR, gamma/delta cells may play critical, and perhaps unique, roles in immune protection at body surfaces.

Mucosal A diverse set of native defense mechanisms is very important
Immunity for protecting against infection at mucosal surfaces. If these native defense mechanisms are disrupted, the individual will have an increased susceptibility to infection at mucosal surfaces.

Lymphocytes responsible for acquired immunity at mucosal surfaces tend to traffic between the blood and submucosal lymphoid tissues, whereas lymphocytes responsible for immunity in the deeper tissues traffic between the blood and lymph nodes.

Antigens that enter through mucosal surfaces tend to induce dimeric IgA antibody secretion and intraepithelial T lymphocytes to defend mucosal surfaces.

Secretory IgA on mucosal surfaces is important for blocking attachment of bacteria, viruses, and toxins to epithelial cells.

Intraepithelial Intraepithelial lymphocytes (IELs) are a population of spe-
Lymphocytes cialized T lymphocytes located within the epithelium of mucosal surfaces.

IELs play important roles in surveillance, homeostasis, and regulation of immune responses at mucosal surfaces.

Leukocyte Leukocytes migrate from the blood into tissues as they are
Trafficking needed to mount immune responses.

Leukocyte traffic is regulated by the expression of a complex set of complementary receptor-ligand molecules on leukocyte and blood vessel membranes.

Lymphocytes may return to the bloodstream through the lymphatic system; other leukocytes generally do not.

Lymphocyte Lymphocytes circulate between the blood and tissues, espe-
Homing cially the secondary lymphoid tissues, in their search for antigens.

▬▬▬ List of Principles — cont'd ▬▬▬

Naive lymphocytes tend to home to lymphoid tissues where antigens and antigen-presenting cells are concentrated. Memory T cells tend to home to the tissues where infection occurs.

Lymphocytes may home to specific tissues where their complementary antigens were first encountered.

Memory Lymphocytes
B and T lymphocytes both respond to foreign antigens they recognize by proliferating and producing, in addition to effector cells, long-lived cells responsible for immunological memory.

Immunological memory is partially due to the fact that there are more cells in the clones that recognize the antigen. Memory cells are more easily activated than are naive lymphocytes when they encounter antigen.

Immunological memory may be life-long or short-lived, depending on the antigen involved.

The Secondary Antibody Response
Subsequent exposure to antigen produces a more rapid and more effective antibody response than the first exposure to antigen.

B lymphocytes undergo class switching to produce antibodies of isotypes other than IgM.

Antibodies produced in secondary responses have higher affinity (binding strength) than do those produced in primary responses

TOPIC 1: Classes of Antibody

Principles

1. B lymphocytes respond to antigen by producing antibodies.
2. There are five major classes of antibodies, each with different roles in host defense.
3. Antibodies protect individuals from disease by inactivating infectious organisms or by helping other components of the immune system to eliminate organisms from the body.

Explanation

The major effector function of B lymphocytes is the production of antibodies. Once they have encountered their complementary antigen and have received the proper costimulatory signals (usually provided by T lymphocytes), B cells proliferate and differentiate into end-stage effector cells called *plasma cells*. Plasma cells differ from naive B lymphocytes in that the cellular organelles that facilitate protein synthesis and secretion are well developed in plasma cells; therefore they are specialized for producing and releasing large amounts of antibody.

Antibody molecules, which are also called *immunoglobulins*, bind to the antigens that induced their production. Antibodies may facilitate removal of foreign antigens from the body, focus inflammatory mediators at the site of antigen deposition, neutralize toxic antigens, and/or prevent attachment/invasion of infectious agents into the body.

All antibodies are not created equal. Antibody molecules can be characterized by their isotype, allotype, and idiotype. Isotype identifies the class of the antibody. Mammals have five major classes of antibodies: IgG, IgM, IgA, IgD, and IgE. Homologues of all but IgE have been characterized in birds, and lower vertebrates, such as fishes, have only IgM. Class-specific modifications to antibody structure are important because they optimize particular class(es) of antibodies for specific immune functions. *Allotype* refers to differences in antibody structure that are specific to an individual or groups of individuals within a species. Any given species has a variable number of forms (alleles) for the genes that encode antibody proteins, but only one form is used by any given cell. Differences that are due to the use of different alleles are called allotypic variations. One or two allotypes may be present in any individual. The differences in allotype between individuals probably are not important for antibody function. The *idiotype* of an antibody characterizes the variable regions of its structure, which includes the antigen-binding regions. Thus the term idiotype is sometimes thought of as somewhat synonymous with the antigen specificity of an antibody molecule, although it really has broader meaning. Healthy individuals have the potential to produce antibody molecules with millions of different idiotypes.

Molecular structure of antibodies

The basic unit of all antibodies is composed of four protein chains—two larger "heavy" chains and two smaller "light" chains. Each protein chain is divided into constant, variable, and hypervariable regions, depending on how much the amino acid sequence in a particular region varies among antibody molecules within an individual or among different individuals. The constant regions are highly conserved across individuals within a species, and to a lesser degree, across species. The amino acid sequence and conformation of constant regions on the heavy chains determine the isotype of an antibody. Antigens bind to small stretches of amino acids located mainly in hypervariable regions, which are present on heavy and light chains. Changes of only one or a few amino acids in these regions can affect the antigen-binding specificity of an antibody molecule.

When the heavy and light chains combine, they form a Y-shaped structure (Fig. 4-1, *A*). Three-dimensionally the chains fold into several globular domains. The chains are stabilized within and between themselves by covalent bonds between sulfur molecules on certain amino acids (disulfide bonds). The area at the branch of the Y is called the hinge region. It is called the hinge region because the area is conformationally flexible, which allows the molecule to adapt spatially as it binds with antigen.

Some of the first research that was done to elucidate antibody structure involved digestion of antibody molecules with enzymes. From these early studies, nomenclature was derived that is still used today. When antibody molecules are exposed to the enzyme papain, the molecules break apart at the fork of the Y to create three molecules (Fig. 4-1, *B*). The forks of the Y form two identical fragments, which are called Fab fragments because they contain the antigen-binding regions. The base of the Y forms the Fc, or crystallizable, fragment, which contains the regions that determine antibody class. When antibodies are digested with pepsin, the Fc fragment is digested into small pieces (Fig. 4-1, *C*). Cleavage between the Fc and Fab fragments occurs in a slightly different

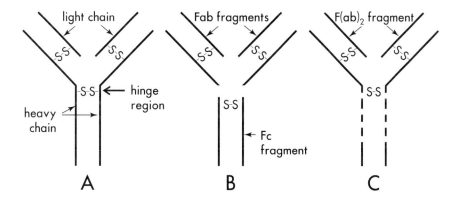

Fig. 4-1   **A,** Structure of basic immunoglobulin monomer. **B,** Immunoglobulin structure after digestion with papain. **C,** Immunoglobulin structure after digestion with pepsin.

site so that the Fab fragments are still joined by a disulfide bond. The combined fragments are known as F(ab)$_2$.

Immunoglobulin G

Immunoglobulin G, or IgG, is the most abundant class of antibody in blood, accounting for approximately 80% of the antibodies in human serum. It is composed of a single immunoglobulin subunit (monomer), and its relatively compact size allows it to penetrate through blood vessel walls and enter extravascular tissues at sites of infection or inflammation. IgG is the predominant class of antibody that is passively transferred from mother to offspring, either across the placenta, through colostrum, or through the yolk (birds).

IgG can facilitate removal of foreign antigens in several ways. IgG molecules can bind to free antigen in circulation or in tissues. If the antigen is an infectious agent, IgG may bind in such a way so that the infectivity, or harmful effect, of the agent is neutralized. Multiple IgG molecules can bind to antigens, cross-linking with other antigen-antibody complexes to form large aggregates that are more easily eliminated from circulation than are small, soluble antigens. IgG antibodies can also activate and enhance the functions of other immune defense mechanisms. IgG that has bound to antigen can fix complement (cause complement to attach to an antigen) via the classical pathway. It can also facilitate phagocytosis of foreign antigens by neutrophils and macrophages because IgG molecules that have bound antigen via their Fab receptors can then bind to phagocytic cells by their Fc receptors. This anchors the antigen to the phagocytic cell so that it can be easily internalized. Also, some infectious agents have properties, such as thick, repellent capsules, that make them relatively resistant to phagocytosis until they are coated with antibodies. The process of coating antigen with antibodies so that they can be phagocytosed is called *opsonization*.

Immunoglobulin M

Immunoglobulin M, or IgM, is the class of antibody that is produced the earliest the first time an individual is exposed to an antigen. It is also produced on subsequent exposures to an antigen, but IgG becomes predominant. IgM is the second most prevalent antibody isotype in blood of domestic animals and the third most prevalent in humans.

Immunoglobulin M is the largest isotype of antibody. It is composed of five linked immunoglobulin subunits (pentamer). Each subunit is larger than an IgG molecule because they have an additional domain on their heavy chains. They do not have a flexible hinge. The five subunits are arranged in a circle, with their Fab segments directed outward (Fig. 4-2). Each subunit is connected to the next by disulfide bonds except for the bonds that close the circle. The final two subunits are joined by a nonimmunoglobulin protein called the *J (joining) chain.*

Because of its large size and relative inflexibility, IgM does not readily leave the bloodstream, so it does not play a major role in immune defenses in extravascular tissues or body surfaces. It is, however, a potent activator of the complement system. The classical complement pathway can be activated by a single IgM molecule bound to an antigen, whereas it takes many IgG molecules to activate the pathway. IgM is also very efficient at neutralizing viruses and agglutinating particulate antigens.

Immunoglobulin A

Immunoglobulin A, or IgA, is the predominant antibody isotype in external secretions, (e.g., milk, tears, saliva) and on mucosal surfaces in humans and most domestic animals. In ruminant animals (e.g., cattle, sheep), IgA is present in external secretions, but IgG performs many IgA-like functions in these animals and is sometimes the predominant isotype in secretions. IgA is the second most prevalent antibody isotype in the blood of humans, but it is present in much lower concentrations in the blood of domestic animals.

IgA may be present as a monomer or a dimer (two subunits) in circulation, but it is always a dimer when present on mucosal surfaces. The subunits within the dimers are connected by a J chain. When IgA dimers are transported to mucosal surfaces, they traverse across epithelial surfaces or through the liver, where they acquire an additional protein called the secretory component (Fig. 4-3). The combined molecule is called *secretory IgA,* or *sIgA.* The secretory component protects the antibody molecule from digestion by enzymes that are present in the intestine and other mucosal surfaces.

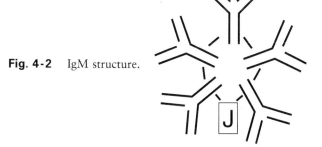

Fig. 4-2   IgM structure.

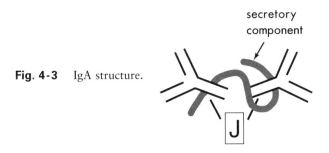

Fig. 4-3   IgA structure.

The function of IgA is mainly to prevent attachment of infectious agents at mucosal surfaces. By combining with infectious agents that are free in the intestine or lung or genital tract, they may hinder the attachment of such organisms to the epithelial surfaces of the body. If pathogens cannot attach to host cells, they are likely to be flushed out of the body without causing harm. Antibodies of the IgA isotype cannot activate complement by the classical pathway, but they can, under certain conditions, serve as weak activators by the alternative pathway. They do not opsonize antigens for phagocytosis, but they can serve to aggregate particulate antigens and to neutralize viruses and toxins.

Immunoglobulin D

Immunoglobulin D, or IgD, is found mainly as a membrane-bound antibody on the surface of B lymphocytes, where it serves as an antigen receptor. It is found on mature, but not immature, B cells. Its absence from immature B cells plays a role in induction of tolerance to self antigens during fetal development. Very little IgD is found in circulation, and it is not usually produced and released during immune responses to most antigens. IgD is a monomer, but it is not as well stabilized by disulfide bonds as are other isotypes. Therefore it is very sensitive to degradation by enzymes found in blood, and it has a short half-life.

Immunoglobulin E

Immunoglobulin E, or IgE, is found in extremely low concentrations in blood and tissues of healthy individuals. Like IgD, it is readily degraded, and it has the shortest half-life of all antibody isotypes. IgE is a monomer, but it has an additional domain on its heavy chain, making it a little larger than IgG.

Immunoglobulin E plays important roles in type I hypersensitivity (allergic reactions) and in immune responses to parasites. Parasitized and allergic individuals have higher circulating levels of IgE. IgE is unique among antibodies in that it has an affinity to bind to mast cells and basophils via its Fc receptor. When cell-bound IgE subsequently binds to antigen, it induces mast cells and basophils to release inflammatory substances. In the case of parasitic infestations, IgE-mediated degranulation of mast cells and basophils attracts eosinophils to the site and exposes parasites to enzymes and other substances that can destroy the parasite, a sort of "reverse mechanism" from normal phagocytosis in which an infectious agent would be internalized by cells of the immune system and exposed to degradatory processes within the cell.

In some animal species, subclasses of IgG and IgA have been identified. Subclasses differ from one another by only a few amino acids in their constant heavy chain regions. Humans have four subclasses of IgG and two subclasses of IgA. Two to five subclasses of IgG have been identified in various domestic animals, as have one to two subclasses of IgA. Certain subclasses may be produced preferentially in response to specific antigens; the significance of this is not always completely understood.

When the host mounts an immune response against a foreign antigen, it is important that the proper isotype of antibody is produced. Protective immunity against many intestinal, respiratory, and urogenital pathogens requires the presence of sIgA at the site of pathogen entry. If circulating IgG, rather than localized sIgA, is produced, the host may not be protected against the pathogen, even though a vigorous immune response is mounted. Also, the antibodies must be directed against the proper site, or epitope, on the pathogen. Protective immunity against viruses often requires antibodies that can neutralize the infectivity of the virus. For example, antibodies directed against the hemagglutinin (HA) protein of the influenza virus are protective because HA is used to attach the virus to host cells. Antibodies against internal proteins of the influenza virus do not prevent host cells from being infected and therefore do not protect individuals from influenza-induced disease.

Related Topics

Clonal development of lymphocytes
Tolerance
Mucosal immunity

Additional Reading

Greenspan, N.S. 1996. Chapter 16. Immunoglobulin function. In Rich, R.R. (ed.) Clinical Immunology: Principles and Practice. Mosby-Year Book, St. Louis.

Tizard, I. 1996. Chapter 13. Antibodies: soluble forms of BCR. In Veterinary Immunology: An Introduction, 5th ed. W.B. Saunders, Philadelphia.

TERMS:

Agglutination	The process of binding antigens and antibodies into large clumps that fall out of suspension. Agglutinated antigens are more easily removed from the body.
Allotype	Classification of antibodies based on differences resulting from multiple alleles of antibody genes present in different individuals within a species. Allotypic differences may be detected as foreign antigenic sites by other individuals of the species that do not possess the same allele.
Fab Fragment	Standard nomenclature for the portion of the antibody molecule that binds antigen. Fab fragments are produced when antibodies are digested with papain.
Fc Fragment	Standard nomenclature for the portion of the antibody molecule that does not bind antigen but through which antibody molecules bind to the surface of various cells of the immune system. Fc fragments are produced when antibodies are digested with papain.
Idiotype	Classification of antibodies based on differences in the variable and hypervariable regions of the antibody, including the antigen-binding site. Antibodies of different idiotypes recognize different antigens. Individuals have the capability to produce antibodies with millions of different idiotypes.
Isotype	Classification of antibodies based on differences in the constant region of the heavy chain. Isotypes are constant among individuals of the same species and are similar between species. Different isotypes of antibodies are specialized for different functions.
Opsonization	The process of coating antigen with antibody molecules so that the antigen is more easily ingested by phagocytic cells.
Precipitation	Process similar to agglutination except that the antigenic particles are usually smaller and soluble.

Study Questions

1. How do the structural differences between isotypes of antibodies adapt them to specialized functions? Give two examples.
2. Which class of antibody:
   - Is produced first in a primary immune response?
   - Is the predominant class of antibody in the circulation?
   - Is too large to readily diffuse into the tissues?
   - Binds to mast cell Fc receptors?
   - Is found almost exclusively on B-cell surfaces?
   - Plays an important role in allergies?
   - Is important for protecting mucosal surfaces?
3. Draw the basic structure of an IgG molecule and label its major components.

TOPIC 2: Helper T Lymphocytes

Principles

1. Helper T lymphocytes respond to antigens by secreting many different cytokines in different combinations and participating in cell-cell contacts that orchestrate cell-mediated immunity.
2. Helper T lymphocytes enable B lymphocytes to produce strong antibody responses to most antigens.
3. Signals from helper T lymphocytes make other leukocytes more aggressive and efficient.

Explanation

Helper T (T_h) lymphocytes are a subset of T lymphocytes that, instead of killing cells or eliminating invading infectious agents directly, participate in the immune response by enhancing the functions of other cells of the immune system. One way that they do this is by secreting cytokines, which are small, soluble molecules used to communicate between cells. They also regulate immune responses by direct cellular contact with neighboring cells, which results in the transfer of regulatory signals through receptor/antireceptor linkages between cell surfaces. The function of T_h lymphocytes can be compared with that of an orchestra director, sending signals to individual instrumentalists (other immune cells) to organize their combined efforts into the most effective overall responses (Fig. 4-4).

The proper cytokine, or combination of cytokines, can induce other cells of the immune system to proliferate, to secrete proteins, or to be more aggressive in their efforts to eliminate foreign antigens. Cytokines

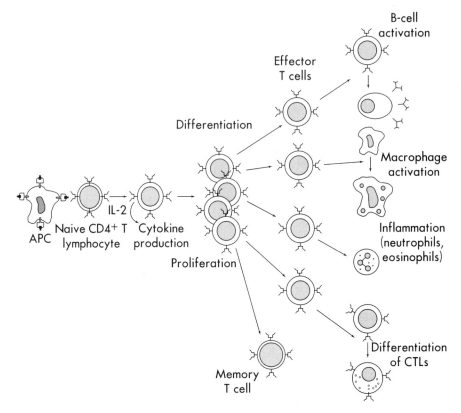

Fig. 4-4   Functions of CD4+ helper T lymphocytes. (From Rich, R.R. [ed.] 1996. Clinical Immunology: Principles and Practice. Mosby-Year Book, St. Louis.)

are not antigen specific; they can affect any cell that possesses the necessary specific receptors to bind to them. Consequently, T$_h$ lymphocytes can regulate the actions of other antigen-specific lymphocytes and the non–antigen-specific white blood cells of the immune system.

Most B lymphocytes require help from T$_h$ lymphocytes to produce abundant antibodies of high affinity. The requirement for T cell help depends on the type of antigen against which the B lymphocyte is reacting. Certain simple antigens with highly repeated subunits in their structures, such as carbohydrates, are T-independent antigens. However, the vast majority of antigens, including proteins and their derivatives, are T dependent. Without the influence of cytokines provided by T$_h$ lymphocytes, B lymphocytes only can generate limited quantities of low-affinity

IgM antibodies. Cytokines, including interleukin-1, -2, -4, and -5, are needed to stimulate B cells to mature into plasma cells and undergo class switching and affinity maturation.

Helper T lymphocytes stimulate many other cells of the immune system to perform their functions more efficiently and aggressively. Natural killer (NK) lymphocytes become more efficient at killing target cells and are effective against a wider range of targets when they are stimulated by interleukin-2. Stimulated NK cells, known as *lymphokine-activated killer (LAK) cells,* are so potent that their potential use in cancer therapy is being evaluated. Macrophages are stimulated by several T_h-derived cytokines, especially interferon-gamma. Stimulated, or "angry," macrophages express more receptors for antibodies and complement, which makes them more efficient at phagocytosing antigen-antibody complexes. Angry macrophages contain more enzyme-laden granules in their cytoplasm, which enhances their ability to destroy ingested antigens. Neutrophils may also be stimulated to up-regulate their surface receptors and enzyme systems by several cytokines; interleukin-8 is an especially specific activator of neutrophils.

Helper T lymphocytes regulate activities of other T lymphocytes. For example, interleukin-2 induces proliferation and clonal expansion of cytotoxic T lymphocytes, suppressor T lymphocytes, and other T_h lymphocytes. Secreted IL-2 also can affect the cell that secreted it (autoregulation), stimulating the cell to proliferate further and to express more surface receptors for IL-2.

Cytokines produced by T_h cells can qualitatively influence future differentiation of the lymphocytes they affect. Immunologists are discovering that, instead of clearly defined subsets of lymphocytes with set functions and set collections of secretory molecules and receptors, lymphocytes within a subset (helper, cytotoxic, suppressor) are heterogeneous. Individual cells within a population may secrete different patterns of cytokines and have different arrays of surface receptors. These differences may be qualitative and/or quantitative, and the differences may influence the specific contribution that an individual cell makes to the overall immune response. Immunologists believe that the heterogeneity in lymphocyte populations is due, in part, to the cytokines in their environment at the time of their differentiation into functional effector cells. Because T_h lymphocytes are responsible for the production of many types of cytokines, their role in cell differentiation can be a significant factor in the type of overall immune response that develops in response to a foreign antigen.

Helper T lymphocytes also regulate other cells through direct cellular contact. Lymphocytes possess a diverse array of receptors on their cell surfaces (Fig. 4-5). The function of many of these receptors was, and for some, still is, unclear to immunologists. However, it is becoming increasingly apparent that several of these receptors are used for direct cell-cell communication among cells of the immune system. Other cells possess receptors that are complementary to the receptors on T_h lymphocytes. When the receptors of these two cells bind, a direct bridge is formed between the cells. Regulatory signals may be transmitted through these receptor links. The communication may be bidirectional; that is, other cells may provide feedback signals to helper cells. Research on direct cellular communication is quite active and the nomenclature system for receptors involved in molecular cross-talk is constantly evolving, but

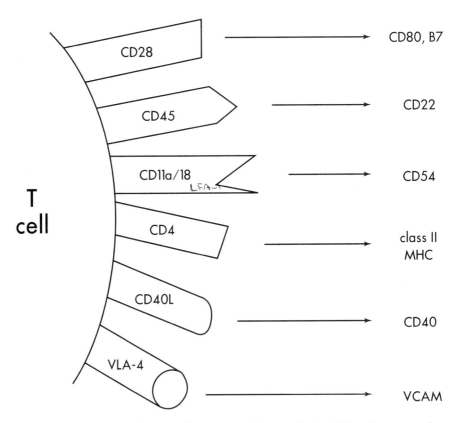

Fig. 4-5   Communication via direct contact between helper T lymphocytes and other cells of the immune system is accomplished when T-cell receptors bind to their complementary molecules (ligands) on other cells. Signaling is very complex because each receptor-ligand pair, or combination of multiple receptor-ligand pairs, has the potential to generate a unique cellular signal. Selected T_h-cell receptors and their ligands are shown.

specific receptors are usually designated by the letters CD (i.e., cluster designation) and a number (e.g., CD40).

It is difficult to make generalizations about the specific effects of certain cytokines or certain receptor linkages because all of these regulatory signals work together to influence individual cells. It therefore becomes important to consider and to appreciate regulation by helper T lymphocytes as a complex and dynamic process, delicately balanced to provide effective immune defenses against infectious agents and abnormal cells.

Related Topics

Cytokines
The secondary antibody response

Additional Reading

Clark, E.A. and Ledbetter, J.A. 1994. How B and T cells talk to each other. Nature. 367:425-428.
Feldmann, M. 1996. Chapter 8. Cell cooperation in the antibody response. In Roitt, I., Brostoff, J., and Male, D. (eds.) Immunology, 4th ed. Mosby-Year Book, St. Louis.
Rook, G. 1996. Chapter 9. Cell-mediated immune reactions. In Roitt, I., Brostoff, J., and Male, D. (eds.) Immunology, 4th ed. Mosby-Year Book, St. Louis.

TERMS:

Cytokine	Low–molecular-weight molecules secreted by helper T lymphocytes and other cells of the immune system that are used for communication between cells.
Helper T Lymphocyte	Subset of T lymphocytes that enhances the actions of other cells of the immune system, either through direct cellular contact or through the release of cytokines.
T Dependent Antigen	A class of antigens, including most protein antigens, for which B lymphocytes require stimulatory signals from T lymphocytes to mount an efficient, strong antibody response.
T Independent Antigen	A class of antigens, usually containing simple repeated subunit structures, for which T lymphocytes do not provide help to B lymphocytes to mount an antibody response.

Study Question

1. How do T_h cells influence the actions of:
- B lymphocytes?
- Cytotoxic T cells?
- Macrophages?
- Neutrophils?
- Natural killer cells?

TOPIC 3: Cytokines

Principles

1. Cytokines are small, soluble molecules that provide a means of molecular communication between cells. There are many families of cytokine molecules.
2. An individual cytokine may be produced by several cell types.
3. Cytokines have multiple and overlapping functions. Cytokines may even induce the production of other cytokines.
4. Cytokines affect those cells that have specific receptor molecules for them.
5. Cytokines in low concentration will produce a local effect and in higher concentration may produce a systemic effect.

Explanation

Cytokines are a group of low–molecular-weight proteins that act as cellular growth and differentiation factors. They can be produced and secreted by practically any type of cell (although specific cytokines tend to be produced predominantly by one or a few cell types), and they may affect other cells or the cell that produced them. The word *cytokine* is a collective term for many families of growth and differentiation factors, including lymphokines, interleukins, colony-stimulating factors, tumor necrosis factors, and interferons. Many cytokines are involved in the orchestration and regulation of immune responses. Some of the cytokines involved in immune responses are produced after antigen-specific stimulation by lymphocytes; lymphocyte-derived cytokines are more specifically called *lymphokines*. However, it is now known that some molecules originally defined as lymphokines may also be produced by other cell types and that other cytokines that ultimately influence immune responses are produced by nonlymphoid cells and even by cells that are not part of the immune system.

Cytokines that are used to communicate between white blood cells are called *interleukins*. The interleukin family of cytokines comprises many different proteins, and additional proteins are still being discovered. The proteins are numbered (e.g., interleukin-1, interleukin-2) more or less in the order of their discovery. Interleukins perform many functions. Interleukin-1 and interleukin-2 have generalized roles in immune cell activation and proliferation. Interleukin-1 is also a potent proinflammatory cytokine that affects many cells outside of the immune system. Some interleukins (i.e., IL-3, IL-5) act as growth factors for immature blood cells. The effects of some interleukins are predominantly directed toward one or a few cell types, such as IL-8, which is a potent activator of neutrophils. Interleukins are involved in the overall regulation of immune responses; IL-12 plays a critical role in determining whether helper T lymphocytes differentiate into functional effector cells that promote cell-mediated immune responses (T_h1 cells) or antibody production (T_h2 cells).

Colony-stimulating factors promote growth and expansion of cell populations, especially progenitor cells. They are named according to the type of cell whose production they stimulate, although some colony-stimulating factors can affect multiple cell lineages. Some examples of colony-stimulating factors are granulocyte colony-stimulating factor (G-CSF), macrophage colony-stimulating factor (M-CSF), and granulocyte-macrophage colony-stimulating factor (GM-CSF). Some of the colony-stimulating factors can also influence mature cells to be more active.

Tumor necrosis factors (TNF-α and TNF-β) were first characterized by their ability to destroy certain types of tumors. However, it was subsequently discovered that the functions of TNF, especially TNF-α, are far more generalized. TNF-α is one of the earliest cytokines released by cells in sites of inflammation, and it can affect many cell types, including most cells of the immune system. Along with IL-1 and IL-6, TNF-α is one of the pivotal factors responsible for the general malaise one feels during systemic illness.

Interferons were first characterized by their ability to interfere with viral replication in infected cells. Interferons-α and -β, produced mainly by virus-infected macrophages and fibroblasts, respectively, bind to as yet uninfected target cells and prevent virus replication from occurring in those cells. Interferon-γ, also known as *immune interferon*, is produced by T lymphocytes and NK cells. It helps to regulate immune responses by stimulating T lymphocytes, macrophages, and neutrophils and influencing the classes of antibodies that B lymphocytes secrete. IFN-γ also influences the type and quantity of surface receptors that these cells express.

Transforming growth factors are a family of cytokines that were originally characterized by their ability to induce reversible phenotypic changes in cultured cells. Transforming growth factor-β (TGF-β) has been well characterized for its roles in down-regulation of immune

TABLE 4-1   GENERAL ATTRIBUTES OF SELECTED CYTOKINES

Cytokine	Produced Mainly By	Main Functions
Interleukin-1	Macrophages and many other cell types	Initiating factor for immune and inflammatory responses
Interleukin-2	Helper T lymphocytes, NK cells	Induces proliferation of T and B lymphocytes; enhances cytotoxicity of T lymphocytes and NK cells
Interleukin-3	Helper T lymphocytes	Induces growth and maturation of progenitor cells in bone marrow
Interleukin-4	Helper T lymphocytes	Stimulates proliferation of B lymphocytes and differentiation of T_h2 lymphocytes
Interleukin-5	Helper T lymphocytes	Stimulates eosinophils; enhances IgA and IgE synthesis
Interleukin-6	Fibroblasts, endothelium, macrophages, helper T lymphocytes	Induces final differentiation and class switching of B lymphocytes; interacts with IL-1 and TNF in acute-phase reaction
Interleukin-7	Bone marrow stromal cells	Proliferation of immature lymphocytes; induces IL-2 secretion; induces formation of T_c lymphocytes
Interleukin-8	Lymphocytes, neutrophils, macrophages	Neutrophil chemotaxis, stimulates release of neutrophil granules
Interleukin-9	T lymphocytes	Proliferation of certain T_h lymphocytes; stimulates mast cells in conjunction with IL-3

Cytokine	Produced Mainly By	Main Functions
Interleukin-10	Helper T lymphocytes	Inhibits production of IL-2/IFN-γ by T_h lymphocytes/macrophages
Interleukin-11	Bone marrow stromal cells	Induces proliferation of certain B lymphocytes
Interleukin-12	Monocytes, macrophages, dendritic cells	Induces differentiation into T_h1 lymphocytes
Tumor necrosis factor-α	Macrophages, lymphocytes, NK cells	Initiates acute inflammatory changes in conjunction with IL-1 and IL-6; regression of certain tumors; enhances neutrophil function; proliferation of B and T lymphocytes
Interferon-γ	T lymphocytes and NK cells	Interferes with viral growth in infected cells; enhances macrophage function; enhances cytotoxicity of T lymphocytes and NK cells; affects antibody isotype expressed by B lymphocytes
Granulocyte-macrophage colony-stimulating factor	Macrophages, fibroblasts	Proliferation of granulocyte and macrophage progenitor cells; enhances neutrophil, macrophage, and eosinophil function
Transforming growth factor-β	B and T lymphocytes, macrophages, platelets	Inhibits macrophage function; inhibits proliferation of B and T lymphocytes; attractant for monocytes and fibroblasts

responses. Contrary to the actions of many cytokines, TGF-β inhibits proliferation and differentiation of B and T lymphocytes and inhibits macrophage function. It attracts monocytes and fibroblasts to sites of inflammation and promotes healing.

The actions of cytokines are multiple and redundant (Fig. 4-6). Every cytokine studied has been shown to affect more than one physiological process in target cells, and several different cytokines may induce similar effects. Under normal physiological conditions, cells are influenced by several types of cytokines at once. It is often the combined actions of many cytokines that are responsible for the observed effects in recipient cells. For this reason, immunologists cannot unequivocally define all of the functions for individual cytokines. General attributes for several cytokines are listed in Table 4-1.

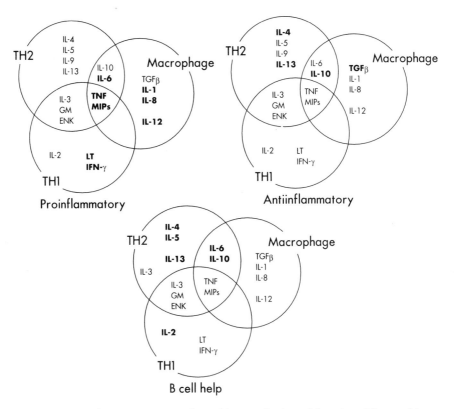

Fig. 4-6   Overlapping patterns of cytokine synthesis and function. The cytokines within each circle indicate the cytokines made by that cell type. Note the overlap between two or even three cell types for the synthesis of a particular cytokine. The cytokines shown in bold letters in each section are those cytokines that are major mediators of the response specified. (From Rich, R.R. [ed.] 1996. Clinical Immunology: Principles and Practice. Mosby-Year Book, St. Louis.)

Cytokines are usually secreted in limited quantities. Therefore, they are usually active only across short distances because they are quickly diluted to substimulating levels as they diffuse into extracellular spaces. This property is important for controlling inflammatory and immune responses because cytokines can often affect many types of cells. Widespread cell activation, away from the site of infection, could be detrimental to the host. However, in cases of severe inflammation or infection, circulating levels of cytokines may rise to clinically significant levels and affect the host systemically.

Cytokines affect those cells that have a specific surface membrane receptor to which they can bind. If a cell does not possess the proper receptor, the cytokine cannot bind to the cell and cannot affect the function of that cell. Thus, the presence of cytokine receptors on cell membranes and the quantity of those receptors constitute critical control points in the regulation of cytokine-induced cellular changes. Receptors for several cytokines have been characterized, and research in this area is quite active. By identifying the receptors, immunologists then hope to identify molecules that can block certain receptors, thus developing means to control inappropriate immune responses or to stimulate responses in immunosuppressed patients.

For example, interleukin-1 plays a critical role in the inflammatory changes that destroy joint surfaces in patients with rheumatoid arthritis. The receptor for IL-1 has been identified, as has a naturally occurring molecule that can bind to the receptor and prevent IL-1 from binding. This molecule is called an *IL-1 receptor antagonist (IL-1RA)*. Clinical trials are under way to see if the administration of synthetic IL-1RA can reduce IL-1 mediated inflammation in affected joints, thus reducing the need for steroids or cytotoxic drugs, which have objectionable side effects.

Related Topics

Helper T lymphocyte subsets
The acute phase-response

Additional Reading

Balkwill, F.R. and Burke, F. 1989. The cytokine network. Immunol. Today. 10:299-304.

Mosmann, T. 1996. Chapter 13. Cytokines and immune regulation. In Rich, R.R. (ed.) Clinical Immunology: Principles and Practice. Mosby-Year Book, St. Louis.

Tizard, I. 1996. Chapter 12. Cytokines and the immune system. In Veterinary Immunology: An Introduction, 5th ed. W.B. Saunders, Philadelphia.

TERMS:

Colony Stimulating Factors	Family of cytokines known for their growth-promoting effects on immune cell precursors.
Interferons	Family of cytokines first characterized for their ability to interfere with viral infection of cells.
Interleukins	A family of cytokines first characterized as molecules involved in communication between white blood cells, although it is now known that interleukins may also affect other types of cells.
Transforming Growth Factors	Family of cytokines first described for their ability to transform the phenotype of cells but which are also involved in the regulation (especially down-regulation) of the immune response.
Tumor Necrosis Factors	Family of cytokines known for their proinflammatory properties.

Study Questions

1. Why is it advantageous for the immune system to have cytokines with redundant functions?
2. Why is it difficult for immunologists to characterize exactly and completely the functions of a particular cytokine in vivo?
3. What determines if a cell will respond to a cytokine in its environment?
4. What determines if a cytokine will have a local or systemic effect?

TOPIC 4: Helper T Lymphocyte Subsets

Principles

1. Helper T lymphocytes may be divided into T_h1 and T_h2 subsets based on whether they primarily induce a cell-mediated immune response or an antibody response.

2. Each subset secretes a distinct combination of cytokines.
3. In the continuum between pure T_h1 and pure T_h2 responses, most immune responses are characterized by a mixture of the two responses.

Explanation

As discussed previously, helper T lymphocytes help orchestrate cellular immune responses by secreting cytokines. Many different cytokines have been characterized, and new molecules are continually being discovered. Individual T_h cells can secrete several cytokines at once, but the types and amounts secreted may vary with the nature of the stimulus and the activation state of the lymphocyte. The pattern of cytokines that is secreted by T_h lymphocyte populations is very important because it influences the type of immune response that ensues. Certain cytokines stimulate cell-mediated immune responses, such as cytotoxicity and delayed-type hypersensitivity. Other cytokines are more effective at promoting growth and development of B lymphocytes, which ultimately produce antibodies. Subclasses of CD4+ T_h cells have been described to differentiate among those cell populations that express different patterns of cytokines. Helper T lymphocytes that secrete cytokines that generally support cell-mediated immune responses are called T_h1 *lymphocytes;* T_h cells that produce cytokines that generally stimulate antibody production are called T_h2 *lymphocytes.*

"Prototype" T_h1 and T_h2 lymphocytes were first described in mice. Evidence suggests that a similar dichotomy exists in humans and other animal species, but the distinction between T_h1 and T_h2 cells may not be as clear in all species. The murine T_h1 lymphocyte response is characterized by the secretion of interleukin-2 (IL-2) and interferon-gamma (IF-γ), with very little or no IL-4, IL-5, or IL-10. T_h2 responses are characterized by IL-4, IL-5, IL-6, and IL-10 secretion, with little or no IL-2 or IF-γ.

Helper type 1 responses are seen in response to viral and bacterial infections and are characterized by enhanced cytotoxicity, recruitment of inflammatory cells to infected sites (delayed-type hypersensitivity), and production of selected classes of antibodies, including those that participate in antibody-dependent cell-mediated cytotoxicity (ADCC). Helper type 2 responses are often initiated in response to parasitic infections and allergic reactions and are characterized by the production of all classes of antibodies, including IgE, and the stimulation of eosinophils and mast cells (Fig. 4-7).

T_h1 and T_h2 lymphocytes probably arise from a common precursor cell. Differentiation of cells into T_h1 or T_h2 patterns of cytokine secretion

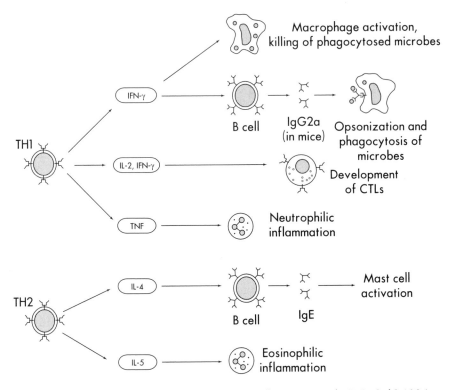

Fig. 4-7   Effector functions of T_h1 and T_h2 cells. (From Rich, R.R. [ed.] 1996. Clinical Immunology: Principles and Practice. Mosby-Year Book, St. Louis.)

appears to occur quickly after an infection starts, probably within the first 3 to 4 days. Whether an antigen-stimulated T_h lymphocyte differentiates into a T_h1 or T_h2 cell depends on the types of cytokines in its environment and the costimulatory signals it receives at the time of differentiation (Fig. 4-8). Interleukin-12 appears to be a critical cytokine in this respect; the presence of IL-12 strongly stimulates cells to become T_h1 cells. Once differentiation toward one subset or the other begins, the immune response tends to continue in that direction because the cytokines produced by T_h1 lymphocytes tend to inhibit T_h2 cell development and/or the expression of T_h2 cytokines and vice versa. This negative cross-regulation helps to explain why clinical immune responses may be characterized by strong T_h1 or T_h2 responses, but usually not both. That is, strong cell-mediated reactions are often associated with weak antibody responses and strong antibody production is often accompanied by poor cell-mediated reactivity.

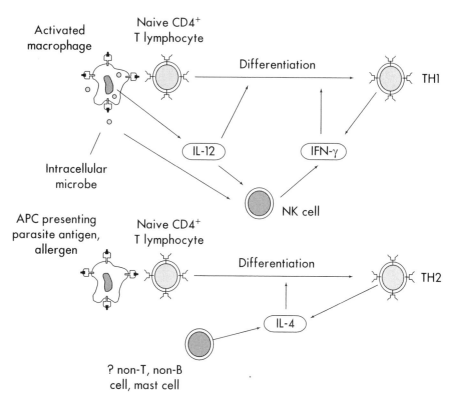

Fig. 4-8   Stimuli for the differentiation of naive CD4+ T cells into T_h1 and T_h2 subsets. (From Rich, R.R. [ed.] 1996. Clinical Immunology: Principles and Practice. Mosby-Year Book, St. Louis.)

Pure T_h1 or T_h2 responses should be considered as polar extremes in a continuum of immune responses. Most, if not all, infections in vivo elicit immune responses with some components of each type. Also, not all T_h lymphocytes within a population express cytokine patterns that fit the definitions of T_h1 or T_h2 cells; such cells are called *T_h0 cells*. T_h0 cells are more prevalent in humans than in mice. T_h0 cells may represent a less differentiated cell than T_h1 or T_h2 cells, or they may participate in a different pattern of cytokine secretion that has yet to be characterized by immunologists.

The tendency for bacterial and viral infections to induce T_h1 responses and parasitic infections to elicit T_h2 responses may be a natural extension of the native immune mechanisms that are activated in early responses to infection. Intracellular bacteria and viruses often infect and activate macrophages and stimulate natural killer (NK) cells. Activated macrophages and NK cells are major producers of IL-12 and IF-γ, which promote differentiation into T_h1 lymphocytes. Some parasites are less effective at activating macrophages and NK cells and instead activate mast cells, which produce IL-4. Interleukin-4, in the absence of IL-12 and IF-γ, is critical for differentiation into T_h2 cells.

The type of immune response that is generated can determine whether an infectious agent is eliminated. Mice that can generate T_h1-type immunity in response to infection with *Leishmania* clear the organism, whereas mice that generate T_h2 responses succumb to lethal *Leishmania* infections. Many of the lesions in the mice that die are due to the inappropriate actions of the immune system itself (immunopathology) rather than to direct effects of the infectious organism. The tendency to produce T_h1 or T_h2 responses is determined, in part, by the genetic makeup of the host. However, immunologists are trying to determine what other factors may be involved in the induction of T_h1 or T_h2 responses so that they might design vaccines that preferentially stimulate the appropriate type of immunity.

For example, immunologists have improved the efficacy of *Leishmania* vaccines by the simultaneous administration of IF-γ, which stimulates T_h1 responses instead of the T_h2 responses that were often generated in response to earlier vaccines. Likewise, immunologists have separated the component proteins of *Schistosoma mansoni* worms and have tested the separated proteins for their ability to stimulate T_h1 lymphocyte responses in vitro. These proteins might be candidates for inclusion in a subunit vaccine.

Related Topics

Helper T lymphocytes
Cytokines

Additional Reading

Del Prete, G., Maggi, E., and Romagnani, S. 1994. Human T_h1 and T_h2 cells: functional properties, mechanisms of regulation, and role in disease. Lab. Invest. 70:299-306.

Fitch, F.W., McKisic, M.D., Lancki, D.W., and Gejewski, T.F. 1993. Differential regulation of murine lymphocyte subsets. Annu. Rev. Immunol. 11:29-48.

Romagnani, S. 1992. Induction of T_h1 and T_h2 responses: a key role for the "natural" immune response? Immunol. Today. 13(10):379-381.

Street, N.E. and Mosmann, T.R. 1991. Functional diversity of T lymphocytes due to secretion of different cytokine patterns. FASEB J. 5:171-177.

TERMS:

Helper Type 1 Lymphocytes (T_h1)	Functional subset of helper T lymphocytes that mediates cellular immunity and delayed-type hypersensitivity reactions. Characterized by the production of interleukin-2 and interferon-γ.
Helper Type 2 Lymphocytes (T_h2)	Functional subset of helper T lymphocytes that mediates antibody production and stimulates eosinophils and mast cells. Characterized by the production of interleukins-4, -5, -6, and -10.
T_h0 Lymphocytes	Helper T lymphocytes that do not fit the strict characteristics of either T_h1 or T_h2 lymphocytes. T_h0 lymphocytes may share features of both T_h1 and T_h2 cells.

Study Questions

1. How do T_h1 and T_h2 lymphocyte subsets differ?
2. How does knowledge of T cell subsets affect design of vaccines and immunomodulatory treatments for specific diseases?
3. What factors influence differentiation into either T_h1 or T_h2 cells?

TOPIC 5: Cytotoxic T Lymphocytes

Principles

1. Cytotoxic T lymphocytes respond to foreign antigens presented on cell surfaces by killing the cells that produced the antigens.
2. Cytotoxic T lymphocytes differ from natural killer cells in that they kill cells in an antigen-specific manner.
3. At least two mechanisms are used by cytotoxic T lymphocytes to kill target cells (the perforin-mediated pathway and the FAS-mediated pathway).

Explanation

Cytotoxic T lymphocytes (CTLs) are a functional subset of T lymphocytes characterized by their ability to destroy target cells that they contact. Unlike natural killer lymphocytes, which can kill a broad range of virally infected or neoplastic cells without prior antigenic stimulation, CTLs destroy cells in an antigen-specific manner. They first must be activated by the binding of antigen-MHC complexes to their T-cell receptors and undergo clonal expansion. Once activated, CTLs are capable of killing only those cells expressing the same antigen-MHC complex. CTLs contribute to the elimination of infectious agents by killing the infected cells in which the organisms reside rather than destroying the organisms directly like neutrophils or macrophages can. CTLs also participate in tumor surveillance and graft rejection by killing cells that express abnormal host antigen-MHC complexes on their surfaces.

There are two main pathways by which CTLs can kill target cells. Both depend on intimate cell-cell contact between the CTL and its target, and after either method of killing, the CTL can disengage, unharmed, from its dying target and go on to kill other cells. The two pathways are called the *perforin-mediated pathway* and the *FAS-mediated pathway* (Fig. 4-9).

The perforin-mediated pathway was the first pathway to be described. In the perforin-mediated pathway, when a CTL recognizes a foreign peptide/MHC complex on a target cell, granules from the cytoplasm of the CTL are exocytosed into the small extracellular space between the membranes of the CTL and the target cell. The granules are secreted preferentially in the direction of the target cell. CTL granules contain several enzymes that can mediate cell damage, but the key component of the granules is a molecule called *perforin*. Perforin is related to complement components C6 to 9. Like the membrane attack complex of complement, perforin molecules insert themselves into the membrane of the target cell, polymerize, and form a transmembrane channel in the target cell. The break in the integrity of the target cell membrane allows ions and water to equilibrate between the cytoplasm and the extracellular space. The net result is an influx of electrolytes and water, which causes the cell to burst.

Cells can be ruptured through perforin-mediated membrane damage alone if enough perforin channels are present in the membrane. However, cells are able to repair small leaks in their membranes by endocytosing the damaged portion of the membrane. In the process of endocytosing the damaged membrane, small amounts of extracellular fluid are also internalized. Target cells under attack by CTLs ingest granzymes and other CTL-derived proteins in the extracellular fluid. Once ingested, these enzymes mediate nuclear breakdown of the target cell. Thus, perforin-mediated cytolysis is a two-stage attack: it causes a primary membrane lesion through the action of perforin and induces secondary lysis of the target cell nucleus should the cell attempt to repair the membrane damage.

The perforin-mediated pathway is a potent mediator of cytolysis, but for many years immunologists questioned whether it was an accurate model because perforin requires calcium ions for polymerization, and

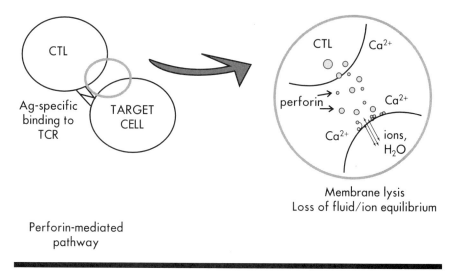

Perforin-mediated
pathway

FAS-mediated
pathway

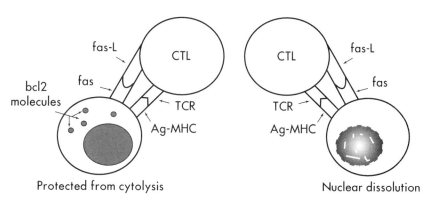

Fig. 4-9 Perforin and FAS-mediated pathways of cytotoxicity.

cytolysis also has been observed under calcium-free conditions. This discrepancy was explained when the FAS-mediated pathway of cytolysis was discovered. FAS-mediated cytolysis does not require calcium, although its effects are enhanced by calcium.

FAS-mediated cytolysis occurs when CTLs, which express a receptor for FAS, bind to antigen-specific target cells that express FAS molecules on their surface membranes. FAS is a molecule that is related to the cytokine, tumor necrosis factor. It is expressed mainly on lymphocytes but also is expressed on liver, heart, and lung cells. The mechanisms that induce cells to express FAS are unclear. When FAS molecules are activated by binding with FAS receptors on CTLs, apoptosis (programmed cell death) is induced in the target cell. The exact mechanism of apoptosis is yet unclear, but the primary event appears to be dissolution of the cell nucleus.

As cells can attempt to protect themselves from perforin-mediated damage, so can some cells resist the effects of FAS-mediated cytolysis. There are certain molecules (e.g., *bcl*2) that protect cells from FAS-derived apoptotic signals. Cells with high levels of *bcl*2 are not destroyed by FAS-mediated cytolysis; however, such cells are still susceptible to perforin-mediated lysis. Interestingly, some viruses render infected cells resistant to FAS-mediated apoptosis.

It is probable that both pathways of cytolysis are active concurrently in vivo. The relative contribution of each pathway depends on the type of target cells being destroyed.

Cytotoxic T lymphocytes also can participate in immune responses through the secretion of cytokines. Like helper lymphocytes, CTLs can secrete a diverse array of cytokines. For example, CTLs secreting interferon-gamma (IFN-γ) can protect other cells from infection by viruses. IFN-γ can also enhance the ability of macrophages to kill intracellular bacteria.

Cytotoxic T cells are usually CD8+ lymphocytes. Therefore, they usually recognize antigen in combination with class I MHC molecules. As discussed previously, antigens that are presented in conjunction with class I MHC molecules are usually those antigens that are synthesized within the antigen-presenting cell, such as viral proteins, and the role of CTLs in the elimination of virally infected cells has long been established. Until recently, however, the role of CTLs in the elimination of cells containing exogenously produced foreign antigens, such as intracellular bacteria, was questionable because such antigens would normally be presented in conjunction with class II MHC molecules, which most CD8+ cells would not be able to recognize. Many immunologists believed that the direct role of CTLs in the elimination of intracellular bacterial infections was minor and limited to the secretion of cytokines. However, it is becoming increasingly clear that CTLs do mediate cytolysis of cells infected with intracellular bacteria. CD8+ cells that recognize class II MHC-bound antigens have been described, and alternate processing pathways in which exogenous antigens form a complex with class I MHC molecules have also been elucidated.

The exact role of CTLs in the elimination of tumor cells and in graft rejection is still unclear. They may lyse these cells directly or mediate their effects through cytokines such as tumor necrosis factor-α. The relative contribution of antigen-specific CTLs and nonspecific natural killer cells also has yet to be ascertained and may depend on the type of tumor cell or graft being eliminated.

In addition to eliminating cells that express foreign antigens, CTLs participate in immune regulation by destroying unneeded lymphocytes. Populations of antigen-specific lymphocytes proliferate and expand in response to antigenic stimulation, but once the antigenic stimulus is removed, excess lymphocytes are eliminated, in part, through the actions of CTLs. The FAS-mediated pathway is probably the major method of down-regulating lymphocyte populations because lymphocytes express FAS and the process by which excess lymphocytes are destroyed resembles apoptosis. CD4+ lymphocytes with cytotoxic properties are probably involved in this type of immune regulation instead of the elimination of infected cells, and FAS-mediated cytolysis appears to be the sole mechanism of cytotoxicity used by CD4+ cells.

Related Topics

The complement system
T lymphocyte antigen recognition

Additional Reading

Berke, G. 1994. The binding and lysis of target cells by cytotoxic lymphocytes: molecular and cellular aspects. Annu. Rev. Immunol. 12:735-753.

Kägi, D., Ledermann, B., Bürki, K., Zinkernagel, R., and Hengartner, H. 1995. Lymphocyte-mediated cytotoxicity in vitro and in vivo: mechanisms and significance. Immunol. Rev. 146:94-115.

Nagata, S. and Goldstein, P. 1995. The FAS death factor. Science. 267:1449-1456.

Podack, E.R. 1995. Functional significance of two cytolytic pathways of cytotoxic T lymphocytes. J. Leukoc. Biol. 57:548-552.

Taylor, M.K. and Cohen, J.J. 1992. Cell-mediated cytotoxicity. Curr. Opin. Immunol. 4:338-343.

TERMS:

Apoptosis   Programmed cell destruction in which a signal to a cell induces nuclear fragmentation and death.

FAS-mediated Pathway of Cytotoxicity	Pathway used by cytotoxic T lymphocytes and natural killer cells to destroy target cells. Cells expressing FAS molecules on their surfaces are susceptible to this type of cytotoxicity. By binding FAS to the FAS ligand on the surface of CTLs, signals are transmitted to the target cell that initiate dissolution of the nucleus.
Perforin-mediated Pathway of Cytotoxicity	Pathway used by cytotoxic T lymphocytes (CTL) and natural killer cells to destroy target cells. Molecules of perforin, secreted by CTLs and NK cells, polymerize in the membrane of the target cell, creating a channel through which ions and water can pass, disrupting the fluid equilibrium of the cell.

Study Questions

1. How do the perforin- and FAS-mediated pathways of cytotoxicity differ?
2. How do target cells resist destruction by cytotoxic T lymphocytes?
3. How can cytotoxic T cells help to control intracellular bacterial infections?
4. How do cytotoxic T cells recognize virus-infected cells?
5. Can a cytotoxic T cell help to control a viral infection in the first few days after the first exposure to a virus? In the first few days after a second exposure to a virus?

TOPIC 6: Natural Killer (NK) Cells

Principles

1. Natural killer cells are a component of the native defense mechanisms that help to control virus-infected and cancer cells without previous exposure to the antigens on these cells. Natural killer cells cannot recognize and attack free viruses or other microorganisms.
2. Natural killer cells are a subset of lymphocytes, but unlike B and T lymphocytes, they do not recognize specific foreign antigenic epitopes and they do not undergo clonal expansion after the first exposure to antigen.
3. Antigen recognition by NK cells is not thoroughly understood, but they seem to kill cells that fail to adequately express normal self antigens on their surface.
4. NK cells look like large granular lymphocytes and use the contents of their granules to kill target cells by inserting pores in target

membranes and by inducing apoptosis (programmed cell death) in target cells.

5. NK cell activity is increased in the presence of specific antibody against cell surface antigens and by interferon and some other cytokines.

Explanation

Natural killer (NK) cells are a subset of lymphocytes that can recognize and kill some virally infected cells and cancer cells. About 5% of the circulating lymphocytes are NK cells. Unlike B and T lymphocytes, they do not require previous exposure to foreign antigens and clonal expansion to be effective. Therefore, they are part of the native or natural defense mechanisms. A single NK cell may be capable of recognizing and attacking cells infected with a variety of viruses or cancer cells. They may play a role in resistance to bacterial and fungal infections by secreting cytokines, especially gamma interferon, which activate macrophages.

Natural killer cells are different from T and B lymphocytes. They mature in the bone marrow and are released into the bloodstream. They do not recirculate between the lymphoid tissue and blood like naive B and T lymphocytes do; instead, they circulate in the blood and home to sites of viral infection. NK cells are larger than naive B and T lymphocytes and have granules in their cytoplasm. They are sometimes referred to as *large granular lymphocytes*. Some activated cytotoxic T cells also have a similar large granular lymphocyte morphology. NK cells and activated cytotoxic T cells use the granules in their cytoplasm for killing target cells.

Unlike B and T lymphocytes, NK cells do not have receptors that recognize specific antigens. They do not rearrange their DNA to generate highly specific receptors for antigen like B and T cells do. They can be distinguished from B and T cells because they do not have surface antibody as do B cells, and they lack several of the molecules normally found on the surface of T cells (CD2, CD3, CD4, and CD8). Natural killer cells do have the CD16 molecule (which is an Fc receptor for IgG) on their surface, which B and T cells lack. Natural killer cells do not undergo clonal expansion after contact with specific antigen like B and T cells do.

The mechanisms by which NK cells recognize virally infected cells or cancer cells isn't precisely known. The evidence indicates that they will kill a cell if they don't recognize a sufficient quantity or quality of normal self antigens on a cell surface. This is in contrast to cytotoxic T lymphocytes, which kill a cell if they specifically recognize a non-self peptide on an MHC class I molecule. One theory on NK cell recognition of target cells is that NK cells detect abnormal expression of MHC class I molecules on target cells. Normal nucleated cells in the body continually express MHC class I molecules on their cell membrane. MHC class I molecules bind short peptides from normal proteins that are synthesized in the cell. It has been proposed that an NK cell is able to detect a decreased number (or absence) of MHC class I molecules and/or the absence of certain critical self peptides within the MHC I peptide-binding groove. If the cell is infected with a virus or is transformed into a neoplastic cell, it may either be induced to decrease the expression of MHC class I molecules or the foreign viral or cancer peptides may displace normal peptides from the MHC class I antigen-binding groove. When an NK cell fails to detect a sufficient number of MHC class I molecules with normal peptides attached to them, this may trigger the NK cell to kill the target cell.

Natural killer lymphocytes and cytotoxic T lymphocytes use similar mechanisms for killing target cells. One can think of them as related cells that complement each other. Natural killer cells seem to be capable of detecting cells that have stopped doing what they are supposed to do (i.e., express self antigens in MHC class I molecules) and therefore will attempt to kill those cells. Cytotoxic T lymphocytes, on the other hand, detect the cells that have started doing something they're not supposed to do (i.e., express foreign peptides on normal MHC class I molecules) and will attempt to kill those cells. A cell that is infected with a virus or has become neoplastic is likely to be synthesizing foreign proteins in its cytoplasm. If these foreign proteins are processed and presented on the cell surface in conjunction with an MHC I molecule, then cytotoxic T lymphocytes should be capable of destroying that cell. If the cells stop expressing MHC class I molecules to avoid killing by CTLs, then NK cells should be capable of detecting and destroying the cell.

As indicated previously, natural killer cells are part of the native defense mechanisms because they can function rapidly on first exposure to virally infected cells or cancerous cells. However, like many other components of the native defense mechanisms, they become much more effective in the presence of antibody or certain cytokines. NK cells have receptors in their membranes for the Fc portion of an antibody molecule. This allows them to attach to and attack any cell that is coated with antibodies. When NK cells utilize antibody binding to attach to target cells, it is called *antibody-dependent cell-mediated cytotoxicity (ADCC)*. When an NK cell recognizes a target cell because it is coated with antibody and destroys it through ADCC, it is sometimes referred to as a *killer lymphocyte (K cell)*. The NK or K cell uses the same killing mechanism whether it recognizes the target cell with the aid of antibody molecules or because the target cell fails to express a sufficient quantity and quality of self molecules.

Certain cytokines can potentiate the ability of natural killer cells to kill target cells. They are especially responsive to interleukin-2 (IL-2) and interferons-alpha and -beta (IFN-α, IFN-β).). These cytokines are likely to be released early in a viral infection, resulting in enhanced NK cell activity to assist in controlling the infection. A natural killer cell that has been activated by interleukin-2 or other lymphocyte-derived cytokine is sometimes called a *lymphokine-activated killer cell (LAK cell)*.

Like other immune cell types, NK cells not only respond to the presence of exogenous cytokines but also they can secrete cytokines that can alter the activity of other cells. NK cells that have recognized a target cell tend to secrete cytokines that are especially efficient at activating macrophages (e.g., interferon-γ, TNF-α, and, GM-CSF). Activated macrophages are more efficient at processing and presenting antigens to T lymphocytes, thereby enhancing the T-cell immune response. Activated macrophages are also more efficient at killing intracellular pathogens that they phagocytose. In this way, NK cells may play a broader role in helping to control intracellular microbial infections.

Natural killer cells use the contents of the granules in their cytoplasm to kill the target cells that they have recognized. They first attach to the target cell, then they release their granule contents onto the target cell surface. They kill the target cell by the same two basic mechanisms that cytotoxic T lymphocytes use to kill target cells. These pathways are the perforin-mediated pathway and the Fas-mediated pathway, which induce the target cell to undergo apoptosis (programmed cell death).

Complete absence of NK cells in either humans or experimental animals is very rare. This suggests that they play an essential function in host resistance. The few human cases that have been described to have undetectable NK cell activity have had recurrent, life-threatening viral infections. This suggests that control of viral infection may be their most essential function. They also may play a very important regulatory function in early stages of viral infection or neoplastic disease by secreting cytokines that may regulate macrophage activity and induce T-cell–mediated immune responses.

Related Topics

T lymphocyte antigen recognition
Antigen receptor diversity
Cytotoxic T lymphocytes
Leukocyte trafficking

Additional Reading

Evans, D.L. and Jaso-Friedmann, L. 1993. Natural killer (NK) cells in domestic animals: phenotype, target cell specificity and cytokine regulation. Vet. Res. Commun. 17:429-447.

Moretta, L., Ciccone, E., Moretta, A., et. al. 1992. Allorecognition by NK cells: nonself or no self. Immunol. Today. 13:300-306.

Seaman, W.E. 1996. Chapter 19. Natural killer cells. In Rich, R.R. (ed.) Clinical Immunology: Principles and Practice. Mosby-Year Book, St. Louis.

Trinchieri, G. 1992. Natural killer (NK) cells. In Roitt, I.M. and Delves, P.J. (eds.) Encyclopedia of Immunology. Academic Press, San Diego.

TERMS:

Killer Lymphocyte   A natural killer lymphocyte that attacks a target cell because the target cell is coated with antibody.

LAK Cell   A natural killer cell that has been activated by lymphokines (lymphokine-activated killer cell).

Large Granular Lymphocytes   Lymphocytes seen in the peripheral blood that are larger than naive B and T lymphocytes and that have granules in their cytoplasm. They are either natural killer lymphocytes or activated cytotoxic T lymphocytes. The granules contain perforin and granzymes used to kill target cells.

Study Questions

1. Compare and contrast antigen recognition by NK cells, B cells, and T cells.
2. How can the response of B cells and T cells to antigen enhance the ability of NK cells to kill target cells?
3. What mechanisms do NK cells use to kill target cells?
4. How can NK cells assist macrophages in killing intracellular pathogens?

TOPIC 7: Gamma/Delta T Lymphocytes

Principles

1. Gamma/delta T lymphocytes may recognize antigen in a manner different from alpha/beta T lymphocytes.
2. Immunologists have speculated that, because of their affinity for epithelial locations and their unique TCR, gamma/delta cells may play critical, and perhaps unique, roles in immune protection at body surfaces.

Explanation

Gamma/delta (γ/δ) T lymphocytes reside mainly at mucosal epithelial surfaces. Gamma/delta lymphocytes are a subset of T lymphocytes that differ from the predominant type of T lymphocytes (α/β) by the protein chains in their antigen receptors. They possess an alternative form of T-cell receptor (TCR), composed of gamma and delta peptides, instead of the classical TCR, which is made of alpha and beta (α/β) peptides.

Gamma/delta lymphocytes were first described in the mid-1980s, when γ/δ-specific antibodies that allowed immunologists to differentiate γ/δ lymphocytes from α/β lymphocytes were developed. Unlike most immunological discoveries, which have been made because of unique immune cell functions or morphological appearance, the existence of γ/δ cells was first described molecularly, based on knowledge of the genes encoding the γ and δ peptides. Ever since then, immunologists have been trying to ascertain why these cells exist and what they do. Much of the information in the following discussion is based on experimental observations, and even though some possible underlying mechanisms for these observations are offered, the reader should remember that, to date, very little about the functional significance of γ/δ lymphocytes has been verified.

Alpha/beta and gamma/delta lymphocytes arise from a common precursor cell. Differentiation into cells expressing α/β or γ/δ TCRs occurs relatively late in cell development. Commitment is made to the expression of one form of TCR or the other; cells expressing both TCRs have not been described. It has been suggested that the γ/δ TCR is a more primitive form than the α/β TCR. Immunologists believe that the genes encoding gamma and delta proteins rearrange first. If the gamma gene of a T lymphocyte does not rearrange because of a "silencer" sequence that prevents it, then the alpha and beta genes rearrange so that the lymphocyte expresses α/β TCRs on its surface.

Gamma/delta lymphocytes have been found in every animal species that has been evaluated. The number of γ/δ cells present in an individual and their anatomical locations vary with the species and age of the individual. For example, ruminants (cattle, sheep) have more γ/δ lymphocytes in the circulation than do humans or mice. Gamma/delta lymphocytes are most prominent in young ruminants and are prevalent both in circulation and in epithelial tissues. Humans have very few circulating γ/δ lymphocytes, and their presence in epithelial tissues is restricted to certain sites, such as the intestine or the respiratory tract. Mice also have few γ/δ cells in circulation, but they are present in almost all epithelia, including the skin.

The appearance of γ/δ lymphocytes occurs in waves. Early in fetal development, γ/δ lymphocytes are the major cell type in the thymus.

These early-appearing γ/δ cells have limited TCR diversity. Part of this limited diversity is because, compared with alpha and beta genes, there are fewer gamma gene alleles to select for rearrangement, but it is clear that certain gene segments are preferentially used by early-developing cells. A second wave of γ/δ cells, which appears early in postnatal life, is more diverse. Immunologists suspect that there may be a developmentally regulated change in how gamma gene segments are selected for use by the maturing lymphocyte.

Populations of γ/δ lymphocytes within some epithelial surfaces preferentially express one or a few gamma gene segments. It is probable that certain lymphocytes home to specific epithelial locations once they are released from the thymus, and immunologists are trying to define specific surface molecules on lymphocytes and the vasculature within epithelia that may facilitate this specific homing behavior. However, it is also probable that some γ/δ lymphocytes, especially certain subsets residing within the intestine, develop within the epithelium instead of the thymus. Such extrathymically derived cells may be subject to different developmental pressures that may favor the expression of certain TCR genes.

Gamma/delta lymphocytes proliferate in response to many bacterial, viral, or parasitic infections and are found in increased numbers at sites of infection. However, the functional significance of these observations is unclear. It has been suggested that γ/δ lymphocytes participate in early immune defenses against invading pathogens, before antigen-specific immunity mediated by α/β lymphocytes develops. This assumption is based in part on the fact that many γ/δ lymphocytes do not appear to recognize antigen in combination with traditional MHC determinants. Freedom from MHC dependence might allow γ/δ cells to recognize antigen more quickly than cells that only can recognize antigens after they have been processed and combined with MHC molecules. Gamma/delta lymphocytes also appear to be activated in response to primitive proteins that are expressed by host cells and/or infectious agents early in infection, such as heat shock proteins. It is likely that γ/δ lymphocytes work in cooperation with α/β lymphocytes, either in unique complementary roles or in "back-up" roles, to eliminate many infectious pathogens.

Gamma/delta lymphocytes can secrete many of the same cytokines that α/β lymphocytes do, but they may not perform helper functions in the same manner that α/β T_h cells do. Gamma/delta cells do not normally provide help necessary for B cells to proliferate or switch antibody classes. However, γ/δ cells may enhance IgA responses by differentiated plasma cells at mucosal surfaces.

Cytotoxic mechanisms used by α/β and γ/δ cells appear to be similar. However, it is unclear what stimuli induce γ/δ cells to lyse target cells. Very few γ/δ lymphocytes specific for microbial proteins have been isolated, but it is possible that γ/δ cells respond to host antigens that are produced in response to microbial infection. Gamma/delta cells are found at sites of graft rejection, but it appears that they may function to down-regulate the response of α/β lymphocytes rather than cause direct lysis of grafted cells. Gamma/delta lymphocytes have also been implicated in tumor surveillance, primarily because they appear to lyse a wide variety of targets in a less restricted manner than α/β cells, but direct evidence for this role is yet lacking.

Antigen recognition by γ/δ lymphocytes remains an enigma. Some γ/δ cells appear to react in the classical MHC-restricted manner, but most do not. Therefore, it is tempting to conclude that γ/δ cell responses are not MHC restricted at all, but it is possible that γ/δ cells are regulated by MHC peptides other than the polymorphic class I and class II determinants that α/β cells recognize. The MHC complex includes many other peptides, several of which have molecular conformations compatible with antigen binding, and certain non-MHC peptides may also be capable of presenting antigen. It is also possible that γ/δ lymphocytes utilize different types of antigen-presenting cells than α/β cells do.

It appears that γ/δ cells may recognize different types of antigens than α/β cells do. Gamma/delta cells are more likely to recognize carbohydrate moieties, heat shock and stress proteins, and superantigens than do α/β cells, although γ/δ cells specific for antigens also recognized by α/β lymphocytes have been described. Immunologists have not yet ascertained how recognition of these different types of antigens may influence the role of γ/δ cells in overall immune responses.

Part of the reason that immunologists have failed to identify clearly the specific functions and modes of antigen recognition for γ/δ lymphocytes is probably because they have attempted to relate γ/δ cell behavior to that of α/β cells, and the model clearly does not fit. Immunologists may need to develop novel experimental approaches to study these enigmatic cells successfully.

Related Topics

Antigen receptor diversity
Superantigens

Additional Reading

Allison, J.P. 1993. γ/δ T-cell development. Curr. Opin. Immunol. 5:241-246.
Cheng, S.H., Penninger, J.M., Ferrick, D.A., et. al. 1991. Biology of murine γ/δ T cells. Crit. Rev. Immunol. 11:145-166.

Haas, W., Pereira, P., and Tonegawa, S. 1993. Gamma/delta cells. Annu. Rev. Immunol. 11:637-685.

Hein, W.R. and Mackay, C.R. 1991. Prominence of γ/δ T cells in the ruminant immune system. Immunol. Today. 12:30-34.

Kaufmann, S.H.E. 1996. γ/δ and other unconventional T lymphocytes: what do they see and what do they do? Proc. Natl. Acad. Sci. U. S. A. 93:2272-2279.

Ojcius, D.M., Delarbre, C., Kourilsky, P., and Gachelin, G. 1994. Major histocompatibility complex class I molecules and resistance against intracellular pathogens. Crit. Rev. Immunol. 14:193-220.

TERMS:

Gamma/Delta T Lymphocytes	A subset of T lymphocytes that possesses an alternative form of antigen receptor that contains gamma and delta protein chains in place of alpha and beta protein chains.
Heat Shock Proteins	Group of proteins, found in organisms as diverse as bacteria to mammals, that are produced by cells in a primitive response to physiological stress.
Mucosal Surface	Body surface associated with mucous membranes, such as the surface of the intestine, respiratory tract, and reproductive tract.

Study Questions

1. How do gamma/delta T lymphocytes differ from alpha/beta T lymphocytes in their structure and diversity?
2. What functions may gamma/delta T lymphocytes play at mucosal surfaces?
3. Where are gamma/delta T lymphocytes found?
4. To what types of antigens can gamma/delta T lymphocytes respond?

TOPIC 8: Mucosal Immunity

Principles

1. A diverse set of native defense mechanisms is very important for protecting against infection at mucosal surfaces. If these native defense mechanisms are disrupted, the individual will have an increased susceptibility to infection at mucosal surfaces.

2. Lymphocytes responsible for acquired immunity at mucosal surfaces tend to traffic between the blood and submucosal lymphoid tissues, whereas lymphocytes responsible for immunity in the deeper tissues traffic between the blood and lymph nodes.

3. Antigens that enter through mucosal surfaces tend to induce dimeric IgA antibody secretion and to activate intraepithelial T lymphocytes that defend mucosal surfaces.

4. Secretory IgA on mucosal surfaces is important for blocking attachment of bacteria, viruses, and toxins to epithelial cells.

Explanation

Protection at mucosal surfaces presents a difficult challenge to the immune system. Mucosal surfaces are exposed to the environment, where they are frequently in contact with pathogens. Mucosal surfaces are moist and often have a high level of nutrients (such as in the gastrointestinal tract and mammary gland) that favor microbial growth. In addition, many of the cells and molecules of the immune system either are not present in sufficient concentration or have difficulty functioning on mucosal surfaces.

Native defense mechanisms are extremely important for protection at mucosal surfaces. One of the most important native defense mechanisms is the presence of normal microbial flora, which helps to compete with, and exclude, pathogens that seek to colonize mucosal surfaces. If the normal microbial flora are disrupted as a result of antibiotic treatment or for other reasons, then pathogens can more easily colonize the mucosal surface. Other factors that help to protect mucosal surfaces include antibacterial cationic peptides in mucosal secretions, the presence of a mucous layer over epithelial cells, the flow of mucus, low pH in the stomach, and an anaerobic environment in the intestines. Coughing, sneezing, vomiting, and diarrhea are all protective mechanisms that help to remove pathogens from mucosal surfaces. If any of these native defense mechanisms is disrupted, increased susceptibility to mucosal infections is likely to result.

An important component of specific immunity at mucosal surfaces is the presence of secretory IgA in mucosal secretions. Secretory IgA comprises two molecules of IgA held together by a J chain and bound to a molecule of secretory component. Secretory component is a protein molecule that helps to protect the IgA dimer from digestion by proteases that are frequently present on mucosal surfaces. The proteases can damage other classes of antibody (which do not possess a secretory component) that may find their way to mucosal surfaces. Secretory IgA is concentrated in the mucous layer covering the epithelial cells and functions largely by attaching to microorganisms and toxins and blocking them from binding to epithelial cells. Blockage of attachment to the epithelial cells will prevent clinical signs from occurring for most bacterial, viral, and toxin-induced diseases at mucosal surfaces.

The lymphoid tissues and cells that lead to IgA production on mucosal surfaces are somewhat separate from those that produce IgG in the plasma. Antigens to which an individual is exposed at a mucosal surface tend to induce the production of IgA on mucosal surfaces. Antigens to which an individual is exposed in deeper tissues, either through systemic infection, injection of a vaccine, or natural exposure, tend to induce an IgM and an IgG class antibody response. Thus, the type of antibody response induced tends to be optimal for protection at the particular site of infection.

For the immune system to respond to antigens present on a mucosal surface, the antigens must cross the mucosal surface so that antigen-presenting cells and lymphocytes can interact with them. Mucosal surfaces, especially the intestine and respiratory tract, have aggregates of lymphoid tissue under the epithelium; in the intestine these are called *Peyer's patches*. The epithelium over these lymphoid aggregates is a specialized epithelium that is capable of transporting small amounts of material from the mucosal surface to the underlying lymphoid tissue, where it can be processed and presented to lymphocytes. These specialized epithelial cells are called *membranous epithelial cells (M cells)*, or *dome cells*. The T helper lymphocytes present in submucosal lymphoid tissues tend to secrete cytokines that induce B cells to become IgA-producing cells. When the B cells in the submucosal lymphoid tissues recognize an antigen, they will proliferate to make more B cells specific for that same antigen and they will rearrange their DNA (class switching) to become IgA-producing cells. These B cells will then leave the lymphoid tissues through the lymphatic drainage and eventually reenter the bloodstream (Fig. 4-10). These B cells will circulate through the blood for a brief period, then leave the bloodstream in postcapillary venules at mucosal surfaces and enter the submucosal tissue. Most of the B cells that originate in intestinal Peyer's patches will return to submucosal tissue in the intestine. However, many of them will end up at other mucosal surfaces, such as the upper respiratory tract, salivary glands, mammary glands in pregnant females, and the reproductive tract. The B cells that home to submucosal tissues will then differentiate into plasma cells and produce dimeric IgA specific for the antigens that were originally encountered at a mucosal surface.

Dimeric IgA produced in submucosal lymphoid tissues needs to be transported across the epithelial barrier and onto the mucosal surface to provide protection against mucosal pathogens. This transport is accomplished by the epithelial cells that line mucosal surfaces. These epithelial cells produce the secretory component protein on the submucosal side of

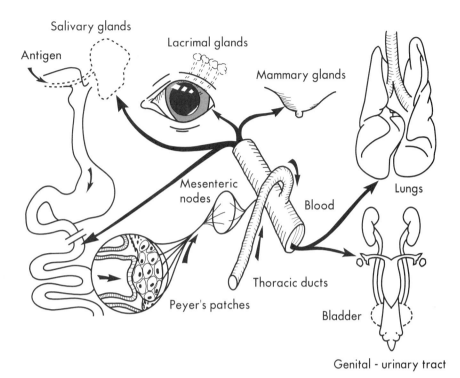

Fig. 4-10   Lymphocyte trafficking in mucosal immunity. Antigens that enter through a mucosal surface (the small intestine in the illustration) must cross the epithelium to be processed and interact with lymphocytes in the mucosal-associated lymphoid issue (MALT) such as the Peyer's patches. After undergoing clonal expansion and class switching, the B cells that recognize the antigen leave the MALT and enter the bloodstream. They then leave the bloodstream and locate in submucosal tissues, where they become plasma cells that secrete dimeric IgA. The mucosal epithelial cells use secretory component to transport IgA to the mucosal surface.

their membrane, near the plasma cells. The J chain of the dimeric IgA binds to the secretory component in the epithelial cell membrane, then the complex of dimeric IgA with secretory component is transported through the epithelial cell and released onto the mucosal surface with the secretory component still attached to the dimeric IgA. The secretory component has a high affinity for mucus, therefore it serves to hold and concentrate the IgA in the mucous layer overlying the epithelial cells, providing a protective blanket of IgA.

Because some of the B cells that originate in the Peyer's patches in the intestines travel to the mammary gland, IgA that is specific for pathogens in the mother's intestinal tract is produced in the milk, thus providing rapid protection to the newborn against pathogens that the mother is shedding from her intestinal tract.

IgA on mucosal surfaces serves to prevent pathogens from penetrating the mucosal surface. However, if a pathogen is successful in penetrating, then the T lymphocyte-directed cell-mediated immune system can play a role in attempting to control these invading pathogens. Mucosal epithelial surfaces contain numerous intraepithelial lymphocytes. These lymphocytes can detect the presence of intracellular pathogens in epithelial cells and pathogens that have been captured by macrophages or other antigen-presenting cells. They can respond by secreting cytokines that activate macrophages, neutrophils, and natural killer cells, or they can destroy infected epithelial cells through cytotoxic activity. The T lymphocytes that serve to protect mucosal surfaces also tend to have separate circulatory patterns from the T lymphocytes that protect from systemic infection, much like the separate circulatory patterns described for B cells that produce IgA. This separate set of T and B lymphocytes that protect mucosal surfaces is called the *common mucosal immune system*. The separate circulatory patterns for lymphocytes that protect mucosal surfaces enable the immune system to provide optimal types of protective mechanisms for pathogens that enter through mucosal surfaces and different types of immune responses for pathogens that tend to produce systemic infections.

Related Topics

Cytokines
Cytotoxic T lymphocytes
Intraepithelial lymphocytes
The secondary antibody response

Additional Reading

Kelsall, B.L. and Straber, W. 1996. Chapter 21. Host defenses at mucosal surfaces. In Rich, R.R. (ed.) Clinical Immunology: Principles and Practice. Mosby-Year Book, St. Louis.

McGhee, J.R. 1992. Mucosal-associated lymphoid tissue (MALT). In Roitt, I.M. and Delves, P.J., (eds.) Encyclopedia of Immunology. Academic Press, San Diego.

Mestecky, J., Abraham, R., and Ogra, P.L. 1994. Common mucosal immune system and strategies for the development of vaccines effective at the mucosal surface. In Ogra, P.L., Mestecky, J., Lamm, M.E., et. al. (eds.) Handbook of Mucosal Immunology. Academic Press, New York.

Tizard, I.R. 1996. Immunity at body surfaces. In Tizard, I.R. (ed.) Veterinary Immunology: An Introduction, W.B. Saunders, Philadelphia. Underdown, B.J. and Schiff, J.M. 1986. Immunoglobulin A: strategic defense initiative at the mucosal surface. Annu. Rev. Immunol. 4:389-417.

TERMS:

Membranous Epithelial Cells	Also called M cells or dome cells. Specialized epithelial cells that cover the surface of submucosal lymphoid tissues, such as the Peyer's patch. These epithelial cells transport small samples of antigens from the mucosal surface to the underlying lymphoid tissue.
Peyer's Patches	Aggregates of lymphoid tissue found underlying the mucosa of the small intestine.
Secretory Component	A protein molecule produced by epithelial cells that serves to help transport IgA across mucosal epithelial surfaces and to protect the IgA in the mucous layer.
Secretory IgA	Two molecules of IgA held together by a J chain peptide and bound to a molecule of secretory component. This form of IgA is found predominantly on mucosal surfaces and is relatively protected from degradation by intestinal enzymes.

Study Questions

1. Describe some of the important native defense mechanisms on mucosal surfaces and speculate on how their impairment could lead to increased susceptibility to infection on mucosal surfaces.
2. Describe the trafficking of B lymphocytes from Peyer's patches to submucosal tissues.
3. How does dimeric IgA get transported to mucosal surfaces?
4. How does IgA on a mucosal surface help to protect against disease?

TOPIC 9: Intraepithelial Lymphocytes

Principles

1. Intraepithelial lymphocytes (IELs) are a population of specialized T lymphocytes located within the epithelium of mucosal surfaces.
2. IELs play important roles in surveillance, homeostasis, and regulation of immune responses at mucosal surfaces.

Explanation

Populations of lymphocytes exist within the epithelia of mucosal surfaces, including the intestine, respiratory tract, reproductive tract, skin, and tongue. These lymphocytes, called *intraepithelial lymphocytes (IELs)*, reside between the basolateral borders of epithelial cells (Fig. 4-11) and play important regulatory and effector roles in immune defenses at mucosal surfaces.

Intraepithelial lymphocytes were first described many years ago, but until recently they were largely ignored by immunologists because experimental techniques to characterize these cells and their functions were not available. Morphologically indistinct from systemic lymphocytes, IELs were once thought to be the mammalian equivalent to lymphocytes in the bursa of Fabricius of birds. However, it is now apparent that IELs are a diverse population of lymphocytes with some similarities to lymphocytes located in systemic lymphoid tissues and some unique features not found in systemic sites.

The number of IELs within specific epithelia varies with the anatomical site, the animal species, and the age of the individual being studied. Intestinal IELs have been studied in the greatest detail; it is estimated that there is approximately one IEL per six epithelial cells in human and murine intestines. Mice also have large numbers of IELs within the epidermis; however, humans have almost none. Intraepithelial lymphocytes have been described for many domestic animal species and birds, but comparative data among these species are largely unavailable.

Intraepithelial lymphocytes are almost exclusively of T-cell origin. B lymphocytes are present in the lamina propria, which is the tissue layer directly underneath the epithelium, but are rarely seen within the epithelium. There are many subsets of T lymphocytes within the epithelium. Many IELs express the gamma/delta (γ/δ) form of T cell receptor instead of the classical alpha/beta (α/β) form. There are many more γ/δ cells in epithelia than are present in systemic lymphoid tissues. In mice, approximately half of intestinal IELs express the γ/δ receptor, and in ruminants, γ/δ cells are even more prevalent. However, as with the total number of IELs, the proportion of γ/δ T cells within epithelial surfaces is highly variable, depending on tissue, animal species, and age.

Intraepithelial lymphocytes can be divided into four categories, depending on their expression of CD4 and CD8 molecules: CD4+CD8−, CD4−CD8+, CD4+CD8+ (double positive), and CD4−CD8− (double negative). Most lymphocytes in circulation and residing within systemic lymphoid tissues express CD4 or CD8, but not both; such CD4+ or CD8+α/β+TCR lymphocytes are also present within IEL populations. However, IELs also contain substantial populations of double positive cells and double negative cells. Double positive cells within the thymus

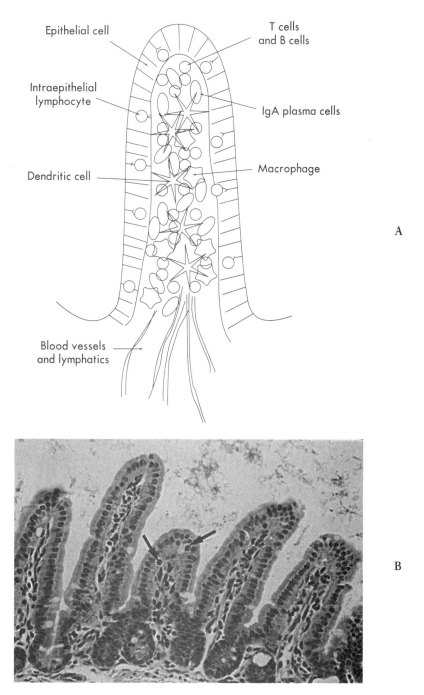

Labels in figure A:
- Epithelial cell
- T cells and B cells
- Intraepithelial lymphocyte
- IgA plasma cells
- Dendritic cell
- Macrophage
- Blood vessels and lymphatics

A

B

Fig. 4-11 Lamina propria and intraepithelial lymphocytes (IELs). **A,** Diagrammatic representation of an intestinal villus. **B,** Photomicrograph of murine small intestine with IELs indicated by arrows. (From Rich, R.R. [ed.] 1996. Clinical Immunology: Principles and Practice. Mosby-Year Book, St. Louis.)

are considered to be immature, and they are rarely seen in systemic lymphoid tissues outside of the thymus. Double positive IEL cells are not equivalent to their thymic counterparts though, and they are considered to be mature, functional cells. Double negative cells within the IEL population usually possess γ/δ receptors and, in many animal species, are considered to be a population unique to epithelial surfaces. Some γ/δ T cells also express CD8, but they express an alternative form of this receptor compared with α/β lymphocytes. This alternative CD8 receptor, called an *α/α homodimer,* is also largely restricted to IELs.

The development of IELs is considered unique in that some IELs probably mature outside the thymus. The concept of extrathymic development is somewhat controversial, but it is generally accepted that precursors of certain IEL subsets, particularly double negative γ/δ cells, migrate directly from the bone marrow to the gut, where they undergo their entire maturation process. Extrathymic development may account for the presence of unique receptor profiles (double positive or negative cells, α/α homodimer CD8 molecules) that do not appear on mature, thymically derived lymphocytes. It may also explain why IELs in certain epithelial surfaces do not have as much T-cell receptor diversity as do lymphocytes in circulation and in systemic lymphoid tissues. Lymphocytes that mature outside of the thymus may be exposed to different antigen-presenting cell populations than those that are found in the thymus, and they may mature in the presence of different combinations of cytokines. Although the selection pressures in the thymus are only incompletely understood, practically nothing is known about development of lymphocytes in epithelial sites and how this site of development may affect final phenotype and function of IELs.

Immunologists are attempting to identify specific molecules that may cause thymus-derived lymphocytes to home to epithelial surfaces. So far, no epithelium-specific molecules have been identified, but it has been shown that murine IELs bind selectively to intestine-associated high endothelial venules, so specific tissue homing probably does occur. Once localized in the epithelium, IELs do not appear to migrate and turn over as extensively as do most systemic lymphocytes. IELs appear to serve predominantly as tissue-specific lymphocytes, where they participate in immune surveillance of their local tissue area.

The functions of IELs are incompletely understood, but it appears that IELs perform many of the same functions that systemic lymphocytes do. Helper T lymphocytes are found within epithelia, and it has been proposed that helper IELs located along the basement membrane of epithelia may provide help to adjacent B lymphocytes in the lamina propria. They may provide help through the release of stimulatory cytokines, or they may engage in limited migration between the lamina propria and the epithelium to participate in direct cell-cell contacts with B cells. IELs also enhance secretory IgA responses by stimulating epithelial cells to produce increased quantities of secretory component.

Intraepithelial lymphocytes help maintain oral tolerance, a state wherein limited local immune responses against orally administered antigens are mounted in the gut while immune responses to the same antigens are suppressed systemically. IELs, in particular γ/δ subsets, appear to induce systemic nonresponsiveness. IELs regulate oral tolerance through mechanisms that are as yet not understood.

Intraepithelial lymphocytes secrete the same types of cytokines as do systemic lymphocytes. Like systemic helper lymphocytes, cytokine profiles of α/β and γ/δ IELs can be divided into type 1, type 2, and type 0 responses. IEL-derived cytokines may affect B lymphocytes and plasma cells, particularly those secreting IgA (as described earlier), T lymphocytes, or epithelial cells. In addition to up-regulating the expression of secretory component on epithelial cells, IELs can also affect the permeability of epithelial cell membranes, ion secretion by epithelial cells, and epithelial expression of class II MHC molecules. Conversely, epithelial cells expressing class II MHC molecules may serve as antigen-presenting cells to IELs, so the interaction of IELs with their neighboring cells should be considered complex and interactive.

Antigen-dependent and antigen-independent cytotoxicity have been observed in populations of IELs. Thymus-independent IELs possess large cytoplasmic granules that contain perforin and granzyme, similar to natural killer cells, and may use similar mechanisms to eliminate target cells. However, nongranular IELs also participate in cytotoxic activities. Target cells may include other lymphocytes or effete epithelial cells. In this way, IELs may participate in maintaining epithelial surface integrity, which is the first defense against invading pathogens.

It is unclear how IELs recognize and are activated by antigen. Some subsets appear to recognize antigen in a manner similar to classical lymphocytes. However, other IELs, especially γ/δ cells, may recognize antigen differently. IELs are not easily stimulated to proliferate, and some seem to be in a state of anergy. Unlike lymphocytes in systemic lymphoid tissues that are relatively protected from environmental antigens, IELs are constantly exposed to myriad antigens. This continual exposure may affect how IELs respond to antigenic challenge.

The study of intraepithelial lymphocytes is still in its infancy, and much of our knowledge of their structure and function is still speculative. However, it is clear that IELs are a dynamic immune cell population that is intimately involved in regulation of immune responses at epithelial surfaces. Because epithelial surfaces provide the first barrier against infectious agents, manipulation of IELs may provide a new avenue for immunomodulation and vaccine development.

Related Topics

Tolerance
Helper T lymphocyte subsets
Gamma/delta T lymphocytes
Lymphocyte homing

Additional Reading

Kiyono, H. and McGhee, J.R. (eds.) 1994. Mucosal Immunology: Intraepithelial Lymphocytes. Vol. 9. Advances in Host Defense Mechanisms. Raven Press, New York.
Sim, G.K. 1995. Intraepithelial lymphocytes and the immune system. Adv. Immunol. 58:297-342.

TERMS:

Double Negative Lymphocyte	T lymphocyte expressing neither CD4 nor CD8 coreceptors. Usually associated with gamma/delta lymphocytes, this population may be adapted for immunity at mucosal surfaces.
Double Positive Lymphocyte	T lymphocyte expressing both CD4 and CD8 coreceptors. Not normally found on mature cells outside of the thymus, double positive lymphocytes are observed within the intraepithelial lymphocyte population.
Intraepithelial Lymphocyte	Lymphocyte, usually a T lymphocyte, located within the epithelium of various body surfaces. This population of lymphocytes may play specialized roles in immunity at mucosal surfaces.

Study Questions

1. What are some of the roles intraepithelial lymphocytes may play in immunity at mucosal surfaces?
2. How are intraepithelial lymphocytes similar to systemic lymphocytes? How do they differ?

TOPIC 10: Leukocyte Trafficking

Principles

1. Leukocytes migrate from the blood into tissues as they are needed to mount immune responses.
2. Leukocyte traffic is regulated by the expression of a complex set of complementary receptor-ligand molecules on leukocyte and blood vessel membranes.
3. Lymphocytes may return to the bloodstream through the lymphatic system; other leukocytes generally do not.

Explanation

Not all foreign antigens are found in the blood or lymph. Therefore, leukocytes in the bloodstream must be able to leave the circulation and enter inflamed or infected tissues so that they can respond to and eliminate foreign antigens residing there. The process of leaving the bloodstream is called *extravasation*. Leukocytes can extravasate through specialized areas of blood vessels, the high endothelial venules in lymph nodes and the postcapillary venules of most other tissues. All types of leukocytes appear to use similar mechanisms to extravasate.

The process of leaving the bloodstream has four stages: tethering, triggering, strong adhesion, and migration (Fig. 4-12). First, circulating leukocytes attach weakly to the lining (endothelial cells) of blood vessels. This phase is called *primary adhesion*. Primary adhesion is so weak that it cannot overcome the shear forces of flowing blood, so most adhesed leukocytes roll along the wall of the blood vessel instead of stopping completely. An alternative behavior of certain T lymphocytes during primary adhesion is called *transient arrest* because the cells temporarily adhere in one site and then release. Primary adhesion is not adequate to anchor leukocytes so that they can leave the bloodstream, but it "tethers" affected leukocytes in one area long enough so that they can sample the local environment. If cytokines or other inflammatory factors that signal a need for leukocytes in the extravascular tissue are present, then the cells are induced to bind more firmly to the vessel wall. The induction process is also called *triggering*. Secondary adhesion, which follows, is much stronger than primary adhesion, and at this point affected leukocytes are anchored to a single site on the endothelium of the blood vessel. The leukocyte then changes from a round to a flattened shape, whereupon it is mobilized to squeeze between the junctions of endothelial cells, cross the basement membrane of the blood vessel, and enter the underlying tissues.

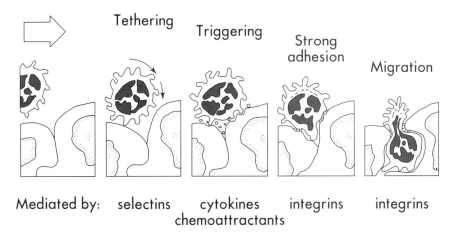

Fig. 4-12   Consensus model of leukocyte adhesion cascade for binding to vascular endothelium. (Modified from Rich, R.R. [ed.] 1996. Clinical Immunology: Principles and Practice. Mosby-Year Book, St. Louis.)

Extravasation is a highly controlled, selective process. On the one hand, leukocytes must exit the bloodstream easily and efficiently when there is a demand for these cells in underlying tissues. However, these cells must not exit randomly because entering normal, healthy tissues would be an unnecessary drain on leukocyte populations and could result in inflammation and tissue damage. Except for lymphocytes, leukocytes that have extravasated cannot reenter the bloodstream to a significant extent.

Immunologists originally thought that leukocytes possessed a unique receptor that bound to a specific ligand (reciprocal structure) on endothelial cells and this receptor-ligand binding regulated leukocyte migration between blood and tissues. Although receptor-ligand binding does play a role in controlling leukocyte extravasation, regulation of this process is complex and dynamic, involving several receptor-ligand molecules, cytokines, and probably other, as yet undefined, factors. It is the balance between all of these factors that ultimately determines whether a leukocyte will leave the bloodstream.

Primary adhesion is mediated by a family of adhesive proteins (adhesins) called *selectins*. Several different selectin molecules have been identified, and they may be expressed on leukocytes or endothelial cells. Leukocyte selectin (L-selectin) binds to specific carbohydrates on the surface of endothelial cells, and endothelial selectin (E-selectin) binds to carbohydrates on leukocyte surfaces. Selectins are expressed constitutively (i.e., all of the time) on the surface of all nonactivated leukocytes, so they are always prepared for primary adhesion. Activated leukocytes quickly (within minutes) shed their selectin receptors. This interesting phenomenon, though incompletely understood, may help to release the activated, bound leukocyte from the endothelial surface so that it can migrate more easily through the vessel wall.

Secondary adhesion is mediated by a family of adhesions on the leukocyte called *integrins*. Important members of the integrin family include molecules called LFA-1, Mac-1, and VLA-4. Integrins bind to ligands that are structurally related to immunoglobulins. Some of the better described ligands for integrins include molecules called *intercellular* or *vascular cell adhesion molecules (ICAMs or VCAMs)*. Integrins are not expressed constitutively on leukocyte surfaces, but their expression can be quickly induced when leukocytes are triggered or activated. Regulated expression of integrins prevents nonactivated leukocytes from binding firmly to endothelial cell surfaces and extravasating into tissues where they are not needed.

Less is known about the factors that control triggering. It is probable that triggering is mediated by various cytokines, which may be produced locally by inflamed endothelial cells or diffuse into the vasculature from underlying inflamed tissues. A family of cytokines called chemokines has been implicated in this role, and their functions are currently under investigation. Interleukin-8 is a trigger for neutrophils. Molecules known as *chemoattractants,* including complement factors (C5a) and bacterial cell wall components, may also provide triggering signals. It is also possible that triggering is mediated through nonsoluble molecules, such as through signaling by as yet undescribed cell-bound receptors.

The ability of leukocytes to extravasate into tissues is important for mounting effective immune responses. Individuals who suffer from leukocyte adhesion deficiency (LAD) are subject to recurrent infections because neutrophils and other immune cells cannot reach extravascular sites of infection. Alternatively, individuals who express too many adhesion molecules are subject to severe inflammatory disorders because immune cells are recruited to an inappropriate degree into inflamed or infected tissues.

Immunologists hope to use their knowledge of leukocyte migration to develop therapeutic strategies for various diseases, including autoimmune disorders and graft rejection. Similar strategies also may be helpful in preventing atherosclerosis, a major cause of cardiac disease, because leukocyte/endothelial interactions have been implicated as a contributory factor in the build-up of vascular plaque.

Additional Reading

Adams, D.H. and Shaw, H. 1994. Leukocyte-endothelial interactions and regulation of leukocyte migration. Lancet. 343:831-836.

Hogg, N. and Landis, R.C. 1993. Adhesion molecules in cell interactions. Curr. Opin. Immunol. 5:383-390.

Springer, T.A. 1994. Traffic signals for lymphocyte recirculation and leukocyte emigration: the multistep paradigm. Cell. 76:301-314.

TERMS:

Chemoattractants	Molecules that attract leukocytes to sites of inflammation. Leukocytes are guided by a gradient of increasing chemoattractant concentration to the source of inflammation. Certain complement factors and bacterial components serve as chemoattractants.
Extravasation	The passage of leukocytes between cells of the blood vessel in order to leave the vascular system.
Integrins	Group of adhesive proteins that mediate strong attachment of leukocytes to the blood vessel wall.
Leukocyte Trafficking	The process whereby leukocytes are recruited to migrate out of the vascular system into underlying tissues.
Selectins	Group of adhesive proteins that mediate weak attachment of leukocytes to the blood vessel wall.

Study Questions

1. By what process do leukocytes leave the bloodstream?
2. What factors play a role in regulating the movement of leukocytes out of the bloodstream?

TOPIC 11: Lymphocyte Homing

Principles

1. Lymphocytes circulate between the blood and tissues, especially the secondary lymphoid tissues, in their search for antigens.
2. Naive lymphocytes tend to home to lymphoid tissues where antigens and antigen-presenting cells are concentrated. Memory T cells tend to home to the tissues where infection occurs.
3. Lymphocytes may home to specific tissues where their complementary antigens were first encountered.

Explanation

Foreign antigens may arise in any part of the body, and lymphocytes must be available to mount immune responses in any site. Also, an individual possesses lymphocytes with millions of different antigen specificities, so there may be only a few lymphocytes reactive against any given antigen in an unstimulated population of cells. To make the most efficient use of available lymphocyte populations, lymphocytes circulate in the blood and lymph, constantly searching for their complementary antigen. They may exit the bloodstream into lymph nodes or other tissues, where they may be stimulated to remain for several days if they encounter antigen, or they may reenter the blood in a few hours to circulate again. Lymphocytes that have not encountered their complementary antigen may circulate through the body as often as every 12 hours.

Lymphocytes begin to circulate immediately on release from the thymus or bone marrow. Unstimulated, naive lymphocytes make up the majority of lymphocytes in blood and lymph, and as they circulate, these cells readily enter secondary lymphoid tissues (i.e., lymph nodes and Peyer's patches [organized lymphoid tissue within the intestine]) that they encounter. The propensity for naive lymphocytes to enter lymph nodes and Peyer's patches is appropriate because secondary lymphoid tissues serve as collection sites for antigens and lymphocytes, and professional antigen-presenting cells capable of mediating lymphocyte recognition of antigens are present in high numbers in these tissues.

Once a lymphocyte encounters and is activated by its complementary antigen, its migratory behavior changes. It no longer enters secondary lymphoid tissue as freely but is likely to migrate to the tissue where antigen was encountered (Fig. 4-13). For example, T lymphocytes recognizing antigens in Peyer's patches migrate preferentially to submucosal sites in the intestine, and T lymphocytes recognizing antigens in lymph nodes draining the skin migrate back to the skin. The migration of B lymphocytes also changes, although they are rarely found in nonlymphoid tissues. Whereas naive B lymphocytes migrate to the follicular mantle of lymph nodes, activated and memory B cells migrate to germinal centers within lymph nodes. This preferential migration is called *lymphocyte homing.*

Homing also increases the efficiency with which lymphocytes are distributed. Some antigens are likely to be encountered at certain body surfaces. For instance, certain bacteria preferentially reside in the intestinal tract, so lymphocytes specific for the antigens of these bacteria are most likely to be needed within the intestinal wall. Therefore, if activated lymphocytes that react with antigens from a certain tissue home back to that tissue, they are strategically positioned and ready to react to that antigen before it can spread through the body.

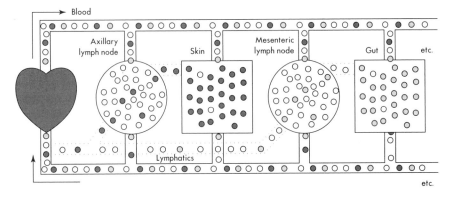

Fig. 4-13 Specialization of lymphocytes depending on their site of primary activation. Solid lines demarcate the blood vessels, and dotted lines demarcate lymphatics. Naive cells (open circles) migrate without preference to all secondary lymphoid tissue. Naive cells activated in skin-draining lymph nodes become specialized memory cells (filled circles) that migrate preferentially into skin. In contrast, naive cells activated in gut-draining lymph nodes become distinct memory cells (stippled circles) that migrate preferentially to the gut. (Modified from Rich, R.R. [ed.] 1996. Clinical Immunology: Principles and Practice. Mosby-Year Book, St. Louis.)

Immunologists have long sought to understand the specificity of lymphocyte homing. They originally thought that the binding of specialized lymphocyte receptors with tissue-specific molecules (vascular addressins) may be responsible for preferential migration to certain tissues. However, identifying tissue-specific addressins and receptors was an elusive task, since the molecules that were identified were too broadly distributed throughout the body to be responsible for tissue-specific homing.

Immunologists now know that the one receptor/one tissue theory is far too simplistic. There are at least five receptor/addressin pairs involved in homing, none of which is limited to expression by one tissue type. These molecules may function in various combinations to mediate binding to a certain tissue.

Activated and memory lymphocytes are very heterogeneous with respect to the combinations of homing receptors they express. The receptor profile of these lymphocytes may be influenced by the activation state of the lymphocyte, the local microenvironment (cytokines, cell-cell contacts) under which the lymphocyte was activated, the type of antigen-presenting cell that mediated the activation process, and even perhaps by the type of antigen itself. Different addressins may be expressed on endothelial cells, depending on the tissue in which the endothelium resides, the activation state of the endothelial cells, and the current microenvironment. A given receptor or addressin also may exist in different forms, with different functional potentials.

In addition to the types of receptors and addressins that are expressed, homing is also affected by the relative concentrations of each receptor/addressin and the presence of many local cytokines that may affect how receptors interact with their addressins. The presence of the appropriate receptors/addressins does not guarantee that homing will take place. For instance, gamma/delta T lymphocytes possess high levels of the receptors necessary to migrate into peripheral lymph nodes. They bind to the endothelial surface, but they do not enter the underlying tissues. Thus, the homing process is multifactorial and dynamic, depending on local conditions at the time of homing.

Because extravasation is an integral part of homing, homing preferences are influenced by all of the factors that influence extravasation of lymphocytes, and because lymphocytes have the potential to reenter circulation, homing behavior is also influenced by factors that act to retain lymphocytes within local tissues. These extravascular influences add another degree of variability to the conditions affecting the migratory behavior of lymphocytes. Extravascular factors have not been studied extensively yet, but they are likely to be even more diverse than the factors affecting cells within blood vessels because of the wide variety of adhesive substrates that may be present in various tissues.

Even though lymphocytes under normal, physiological conditions home preferentially to certain tissues, these preferences can be overridden in cases of severe inflammation. In such instances, high levels of circulating inflammatory cytokines can alter the "normal" pattern of addressin expression in an affected vascular bed. It has been shown that homing specificity is reduced during severe inflammation so that a larger number of lymphocytes can be recruited to the inflamed area. This may serve to broaden the spectrum of potential effector cells in areas of severe need.

Related Topics

The lymphoid system
Mucosal immunity

Additional Reading

Jutila, M.A. 1994. Function and regulation of leukocyte homing receptors. J. Leukoc. Biol. 55:133-140.
Mackay, C.R. 1993. Homing of naive, memory and effector lymphocytes. Curr. Opin. Immunol. 5:423-427.

Picker, L.J. 1994. Control of lymphocyte homing. Curr. Opin. Immunol. 6:394-406.

TERMS:

Addressins	Molecules expressed on blood vessel endothelia that mediate tissue-specific homing of lymphocytes.
Lymphocyte Homing	Preferential migration of activated lymphocytes back to the tissue where their complementary antigen was first encountered.

Study Questions

1. What factors influence homing behavior of lymphocytes?
2. How might homing serve to increase the efficiency of immune responses?

TOPIC 12: Memory Lymphocytes

Principles

1. B and T lymphocytes both respond to foreign antigens they recognize by proliferating and producing, in addition to effector cells, long-lived cells responsible for immunological memory.
2. Immunological memory is partially due to the fact that there are more cells in the clones that recognize the antigen.
3. Memory cells are more easily activated than are naive lymphocytes when they encounter antigen.
4. Immunological memory may be lifelong or short-lived, depending on the antigen involved.

Explanation

It has been well known for centuries that individuals who survive an infectious disease tend not to become as ill, or may not become ill at all, when exposed to the same infectious agent a second time. The immune system remembers antigens that it has encountered before, and it is better prepared to react against such antigens on subsequent exposures. Such is the concept of immunological memory, and for years immunologists assumed that there must be a long-lived population of unique lymphocytes that mediate this antigen-specific recall phenomenon. Recent research, though, has drawn many of those original assumptions into question. There probably is no unique memory cell population; lymphocytes acting as memory cells share many features with naive and effector lymphocytes. The life span of memory cells is uncertain, and they may have a turnover rate more rapid than other lymphocytes. Perhaps most important, the factors that regulate the establishment and maintenance of immunological memory are yet unclear.

Features of memory lymphocytes

Originally, memory lymphocytes were believed to be small, nondescript cells residing in the recirculating pool of lymphocytes. As immunological identification techniques improved, immunologists began to search for phenotypic markers (structural features) on lymphocytes that would identify them as memory cells. To date, they have been unable to describe any molecules that are expressed uniquely and irreversibly by memory cells. The surface molecule CD45 has been proposed as a memory marker for T lymphocytes. Naive T cells express a high–molecular-weight form of CD45, called *CD45RA*. After these cells are activated, they begin to express a low–molecular-weight form, called *CD45RO*. Unfortunately, CD45RO+ cells do not remain in circulation for a long time, which has led immunologists to speculate that, if memory cells are indeed long lived, CD45RO expression may be transient. Cells acting as memory cells, but not expressing CD45RO, have also been described, so this marker has not proved to be a reliable indicator of memory cell status.

Molecular markers for memory B cells are even less clear. Most memory B cells probably express surface-bound immunoglobulin of isotypes other than IgM (which assumes they have been activated to undergo class switching). They may also express high levels of molecules called heat stable antigen and CD44, but this is still speculative.

It is probable that memory cells cannot be identified based on phenotype alone. They share many molecular features with naive and effector lymphocytes, and they may undergo phenotypic changes as they mature and age. They also are capable of secreting a wide variety of cytokines, including those associated with T_h1 and T_h2 profiles, so they cannot be identified by their cytokine secretion patterns. Ideally, memory cells should be identified through a combination of phenotype, activation status, and an analysis of their function.

The lineage of memory cells is also controversial. It is uncertain whether memory cells develop from common precursors with effector cells or if they arise from a different precursor. There seems to be more agreement that memory B cells arise separately from plasma cells than that memory T cells arise from precursors separate from helper and cytotoxic T cells, but even this hypothesis is subject to conflicting experimental evidence.

Life span of memory lymphocytes

The life span of memory lymphocytes is uncertain. Memory could be maintained by a resting population of long-lived cells or by a population of short-lived cells that actively divide. Part of the difficulty in determining the life span of memory cells lies in the difficulty in identifying exactly what type of lymphocyte a memory cell is. As a population, mature circulating T lymphocytes have a long, perhaps indefinite, life span, but the relative life spans of naive and memory cells within the circulating pool have been difficult to ascertain. Naive lymphocytes appear to remain in circulation for long periods, but recent experimental evidence suggests that memory cells may experience rapid turnover.

Factors that influence the maintenance and duration of immunological memory

It has been established that the duration of clinically significant levels of immunological memory varies, depending on the infectious agent involved. For example, humans who have recovered from chickenpox are usually immune from clinical disease for life. However, immunity to diseases such as tetanus or influenza requires periodic boosters of antigen to maintain adequate memory responses. Several factors are probably involved in establishing and maintaining memory, including the physical properties of the antigen, route of exposure, antigenic dose, frequency of exposure, and persistence of the antigen in the host (Fig. 4-14).

One of the variables that has received considerable attention in recent years is the need for persistent antigenic stimulation to maintain immunological memory. Some memory responses appear to last indefinitely,

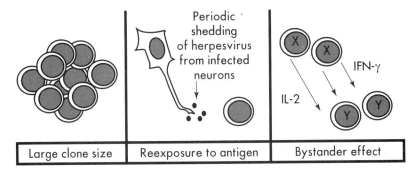

Fig. 4-14   Factors that may enhance duration of immunological memory. Bystander effect occurs when lymphocytes specific for a different antigen are activated to produce stimulatory cytokines, which, when released, can stimulate neighboring cells in a nonspecific manner.

even though the immune individual is not reexposed to the inciting antigen and the antigen cannot be isolated from the host individual, which suggests that memory can be maintained in the absence of antigen. However, recent experimental evidence suggests that many memory responses do depend on recurrent antigenic stimulation, even though the source of the antigenic stimulation may not be readily apparent.

In the case of certain viral diseases, such as chickenpox, direct antigenic restimulation seems plausible because the causative virus (herpesvirus) is known to persist in a latent (inactive) form in nervous tissues throughout an individual's life. Activation of very small amounts of such viruses may be enough to provide the necessary antigenic stimulus to maintain memory even though the host may not experience any overt signs of disease when this virus is released.

For other diseases in which the inciting infectious agent is completely cleared from the host, the source of antigenic restimulation is less clear. Processed antigens that have bound to the surface of certain antigen-presenting cells, such as follicular dendritic cells within lymph nodes, may be retained for long periods (perhaps months to a year), and these antigenic fragments may serve to maintain memory cells. It also has been suggested that memory may be maintained through stimulation by cross-reacting environmental antigens or by bystander effects. Under a bystander effect, lymphocytes responding to an unrelated antigen secrete cytokines, which may affect nearby unrelated lymphocytes (bystanders) in a non–antigen-specific manner. It is possible that such cytokine stimulation may be sufficient to maintain memory cells. It also has been suggested that the need for antigenic persistence may change as memory cells mature. "Early" memory cells may need restimulation, but "late" memory cells may not.

Regardless of whether persistent antigenic stimulation is an absolute requirement for memory maintenance, it is apparent that recurrent antigenic stimulation may serve to enhance the magnitude of many memory responses. It is this concept that is more clinically relevant, especially to vaccine manufacturers seeking to develop effective and long-lasting vaccines.

The underlying factors affecting duration of memory may be related to the size of the original clonal lymphocyte burst. The larger the size of the reactive lymphocyte pool at the end of primary antigenic stimulation, the longer the memory response may last. It is also possible that basal levels of memory cells may be maintained by homeostatic mechanisms other than antigen-specific stimulation, such as circulating hormones and growth factors and nonspecific stimulatory lymphocyte products. This possibility is supported by the fact that the memory lymphocyte pools reactive against many different viruses are quantitatively similar, despite differences in antigen dose and frequency of reexposure.

Functional state of memory lymphocytes

Memory lymphocytes appear to be a functionally resting population of cells. Like naive lymphocytes, they must be activated before they can participate in immune responses to antigen. The activation requirements for memory cells are less stringent than those for naive lymphocytes, which may allow memory lymphocytes to react more quickly and efficiently to an antigenic stimulus than naive cells.

Related Topics

Costimulatory signals for lymphocytes
The secondary antibody response

Additional Reading

Bradley, L.M., Croft, M., and Swain, S.L. 1993. T-cell memory: new perspectives. Immunol. Today. 14:197-199.

Gray, D. 1994. Regulation of immunological memory. Curr. Opin. Immunol. 6:425-430.

Lau, L.L., Jamieson, B.D., Somasundaram, T., and Ahmed, R. 1994. Cytotoxic T-cell memory without antigen. Nature. 369:648-652.

Mackay, C.R. 1993. Immunological memory. Adv. Immunol. 53:217-265.

Sprent, J. and Tough, D.F. 1994. Lymphocyte lifespan and memory. Science. 265:1395-1400.

TERMS:

Immunological Memory	The enhanced immune response that is generated on second and subsequent exposures to a particular antigen. Memory responses are quicker and stronger than initial immune responses to an antigen.
Memory Lymphocyte	Previously activated lymphocytes, currently in a resting state, that can mediate memory immune responses when reactivated by antigen.

Study Questions

1. How might the pathogenesis of a particular infectious disease affect whether long-term immunity is established after recovery from the disease?

2. What is known about distinctive characteristics of memory B or T lymphocytes?
3. What factors may influence the duration of immunological memory?

TOPIC 13: The Secondary Antibody Response

Principles

1. Subsequent exposure to antigen produces a more rapid and more effective antibody response than the first exposure to antigen.
2. B lymphocytes undergo class switching to produce antibodies of isotypes other than IgM.
3. Antibodies produced in secondary responses have higher affinity (binding strength) than do those produced in primary responses.

Explanation

On initial exposure to antigen, resting naive B lymphocytes are activated and induced to proliferate. They are then transformed so that they can efficiently produce large quantities of immunoglobulins (antibody molecules). The transformed cells are called *plasma cells*. Antigen-specific antibodies are first detected in serum about 7 to 10 days after initial antigen exposure. Most of the antibodies in a primary response are of the IgM isotype.

On subsequent exposures to the same antigen, antibody responses are qualitatively and quantitatively different from the primary response. Antibodies are detected in the serum much more quickly, about 3 to 5 days after exposure. The predominant antibody isotype present in serum is IgG, but all isotypes may be represented. Furthermore, the average affinity (strength with which antibody binds to antigen) of the antibodies produced in secondary responses is higher than that associated with the primary response. A secondary response is also called an *anamnestic response*.

Several immunological events occur to account for these changes in the character of an antibody response: (1) clonal expansion of antigen-specific lymphocytes, (2) reduced requirements for activation of memory lymphocytes, (3) antibody class switching, and (4) affinity maturation of the antibody response.

Secondary and subsequent immune responses to the same antigen are more rapid and larger in magnitude than the primary response because they have larger antigen-specific cell populations from which to effect responses. In the immunologically naive individual, only a few lymphocytes are reactive against any given antigen. However, when the individual first encounters a particular antigen, lymphocytes reactive against that antigen will proliferate to form large populations of identical daughter cells. Many of these cells develop into plasma cells and produce antibodies until the antigen is eliminated, at which time they die. Other cells from the expanded population become memory cells, which remain in an individual for an undetermined length of time, ready to react against future challenges from the same antigen. The size of the memory cell population is somewhat proportional to how recently an antigen has been encountered. Antigen-specific memory populations tend to dwindle if a particular antigen is not encountered for long periods, but memory populations are usually larger than the original naive lymphocyte population for a given antigen. The larger base population allows an individual to produce larger quantities of antibodies in less time because lymphocytes do not have to undergo as many cell divisions to achieve a critical number of plasma cells.

Secondary immune responses are also stronger and quicker because it takes less costimulation to activate memory cells than it does to activate lymphocytes that are recognizing antigen for the first time. Recognition of antigen alone is not sufficient to activate naive lymphocytes. They must also receive additional stimulatory signals, which may be transmitted through cell-cell contacts with antigen-presenting cells or through cytokines. Memory cells appear to require fewer costimulatory signals in addition to antigen-specific signals; in some instances, antigen recognition alone may be sufficient for activation. Memory cells are also capable of recognizing antigen presented on a wider variety of antigen-presenting cells than are naive lymphocytes. The reduced need for specific co-stimuli and the ability to recognize antigen presented in more diverse cell contexts allow memory cells to activate more quickly and more easily than naive lymphocytes in response to an antigenic challenge.

Antibody class switching

Individual B lymphocytes are capable of producing antibodies of only one isotype or class (in addition to IgD) at a time. The first isotype expressed by B cells is IgM, hence the reason that primary antibody responses are dominated by IgM antibodies. However, the genes responsible for antibody isotype can undergo a switching event wherein the gene segment encoding the IgM isotype is replaced by a gene segment encoding the IgG, IgA, or IgE isotype (Fig. 4-15). The plasma cell that then develops from that B cell produces antibodies with the original antigen specificity but with a different isotype.

Class switching is largely restricted to antibody responses against T-cell–dependent antigens (i.e., most protein antigens). All (primary and

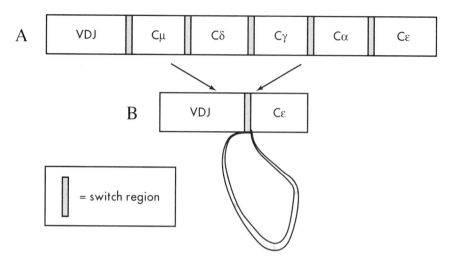

Fig. 4-15   Plasma cells can alter the isotype of antibody that they produce by undergoing class switching. The constant region of the gene encoding the immuno-globulin heavy chain contains sequence information for all isotypes, and the isotype-specific sequence adjacent to the VDJ segment is the one that is tran-scribed. When a plasma cell switches to an isotype other than IgM, the DNA en-coding intervening isotypes is excised at special sites called switching regions. A new isotype sequence is then joined with the VDJ segment for transcription.

secondary) antibody responses against T-independent antigens (i.e., some carbohydrates and molecules with repeating structural units) are pre-dominantly IgM responses, although it has been shown recently that a limited amount of class switching does occur in response to these antigens. Class switching is important to diversify the antibody response and/or to direct its actions because each antibody isotype has certain effector functions (e.g., opsonization, agglutination, protection of muco-sal surfaces) for which it is most efficient.

Class switching requires the presence of cytokines and specific cell-cell contacts. Several cytokines have been implicated in class switching. Transforming growth factor-beta appears to induce switching to isotypes IgA and IgG2b. Interleukin-4 promotes switching to IgE and IgG1, and interferon-gamma enhances switching to IgG2a and IgG3. Other cyto-kines, such as interleukins-1, -2, and -6, promote B cell maturation in general and enhance antibody production by cells that have undergone class switching.

Cytokines alone, however, are not sufficient to initiate class switch-ing. Specific cell-cell contacts are required, and the CD40 molecule appears to play a critical role in this function. CD40 molecules on the surface of B lymphocytes bind with CD40 ligands (receptors) found on activated T lymphocytes. When CD40 binds to its ligand in the presence of appropriate cytokines, signals are transmitted into the B cell that permit it to switch antibody classes. The exact mechanism of CD40-induced class switching is still unclear. Other B-cell activators may also mediate cellular signaling similar to CD40, and these activators may be responsible for the limited class switching seen in the absence of T lymphocytes, but these possible alternative mechanisms are unclear.

Affinity maturation of antibody responses

Antibodies may bind to their complementary antigens with different strengths or affinities. Beyond a certain threshold affinity, which is necessary to activate naive B lymphocytes to proliferate and mature, the antibodies produced by different lymphocyte clones may possess a range of affinities. However, as an antibody response matures, the average affinity with which antigen-specific antibodies bind to their antigen increases (Fig. 4-16). The increase in affinity occurs by a process called *affinity maturation,* and it is important because high-affinity antibodies bind more efficiently to their target antigens.

Affinity maturation takes place within the germinal centers of lymph nodes and is accomplished through repeating cycles of genetic mutation and selection. Germinal centers are composed of centrally located dark

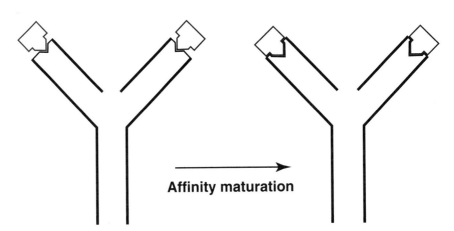

Affinity maturation

Fig. 4-16   Affinity maturation is the process by which the genes encoding antibody molecules undergo mutations that change their antigen-binding regions. When the mutations alter the sequence and conformation of the antibody so that it binds its antigen more closely and with greater strength (affinity), the cells producing these antibodies of high affinity are selected for further growth and expansion.

zones, which contain densely packed, actively dividing B lymphocytes, and outer light zones, where lymphocytes interact with antigen-presenting cells. Activated B lymphocytes accumulate in the dark zone during antigen-dependent expansion of B cell clones. As they divide, genetic mutations occur at a high rate within the DNA of the lymphocyte. The factors that facilitate this enhanced mutational activity are unclear, but such high mutational rates appear to be confined to B lymphocytes within the germinal center.

The mutations that are introduced into lymphocyte DNA are random, so many of them will cause the B cell to produce nonfunctional antibodies. Others may occur in sites that alter the antigenic specificity of the antibody. Only a very few mutations occur in sites that preserve the functionality and antigen specificity of an antibody while changing its affinity for antigen, and fewer yet actually serve to increase affinity. Therefore, there is a selection process that allows cells producing antibody with increased affinity to live while leaving undesirable mutants to die. This selection process takes place in the light zone. Follicular dendritic cells, which are a powerful type of antigen-presenting cell, are abundant in the light zone, and they interact with cell-bound antibodies on the newly mutated B cells. Those B cells that are most able to bind their complementary antigen presented on the follicular dendritic cells are selected for further proliferation and differentiation into plasma cells and memory cells. Those B cells that cannot compete because they do not bind antigen as tightly are eliminated. It may take several individual mutations to create an antibody with increased affinity. B lymphocytes with as many as nine different mutations have been identified; the mutations appear to occur sequentially rather than simultaneously.

Affinity maturation is evident during the second week after antigen exposure. Germinal center development peaks about 2 weeks after exposure and starts to decline about 4 weeks after exposure unless the antigen remains in the host to cause persistent stimulation.

Related Topics

The lymphoid system
Clonal development of lymphocytes
Costimulatory signals for lymphocytes
Classes of antibody

Additional Reading

Berek, C. and Ziegner, M. 1993. The maturation of the immune response. Immunol. Today. 14:400-404.

Kepler, T.B. and Perelson, A.S. 1993. Cyclic re-entry of germinal center B cells and the efficiency of affinity maturation. Immunol. Today. 14:412-415.

Nossal, G.J.V. 1992. The molecular and cellular basis of affinity maturation in the antibody response. Cell. 68:1-2.

Snapper, C.M. and Mond, J.J. 1993. Towards a comprehensive view of immunoglobulin class switching. Immunol. Today. 14:15-17.

TERMS:

Affinity Maturation	Process whereby the average strength (affinity) with which a population of antibodies binds to its complementary antigen is increased. Affinity maturation occurs by a series of mutation and selection events; lymphocytes with mutations in their immunoglobulin genes that serve to increase the affinity of antibodies produced from them are selected for expansion.
Anamnestic Response	Memory response.
Class Switching	Rearrangement of DNA encoding antibody isotype so that antibodies of an isotype other than IgM are produced.

Study Questions

1. How does antibody class switching occur?
2. What is the purpose of affinity maturation?
3. Why is class switching important for efficient antibody responses at mucosal surfaces?
4. How does activation of memory B lymphocytes by antigen differ from activation of naive B lymphocytes?
5. What role do T lymphocytes play in:
   - clonal expansion of B lymphocytes?
   - antibody class switching?
   - affinity maturation?

CHAPTER 5

Clinical Immunology

In this chapter the principles of basic immunology are applied to help explain a number of clinically important conditions and situations. The immune system is essential for protecting individuals from disease. If the immune system is defective for any reason, the individual is likely to suffer chronic or life-threatening infectious diseases. Conversely, if the immune system reacts too aggressively to foreign antigens that are relatively harmless, or if it reacts against self antigens, the immune response itself may cause mild to severe clinical signs or even death.

List of Principles

Autoimmunity   An autoimmune state occurs when an individual's immune system ceases to tolerate certain self antigens and mounts an immune response to eliminate those antigens.

Autoimmunity may be generalized or organ specific.

Many factors contribute to the onset of autoimmune disease, including the genetic background of the affected individual and prior exposure to related antigens.

Transplantation   Transplanted tissues may be attacked and rejected by the immune system if the molecules on the cell surfaces of the transplanted tissue are antigenically different from those of the host.

Matching the MHC antigens of donor and recipient tissues before transplantation reduces the incidence of graft rejection.

Continued

149

List of Principles — cont'd

Graft vs. host disease, in which the lymphocytes in the donor tissue attack the recipient, is a special type of transplantation reaction that may occur in severely immunocompromised individuals.

Psychoneuro-immunology The immune system, the nervous system, and the endocrine system influence one another.

The nervous system may influence the immune system through direct innervation of lymphoid tissues or through the release of neurotransmitter molecules.

Stress affects the quality and magnitude of immune responses.

Several hormones are capable of influencing immune function.

Immuno-deficiency Many factors, including genetic defects, stress, viral infection, toxins, cancer, and old age can lead to defects in immune function.

Individuals with severe immunodeficiencies tend to have severe recurrent infections with unusual or opportunistic pathogens.

The characteristics of a recurrent infectious process may give clues as to the type of immunodeficiency by which an individual is affected.

Hypersensi-tivities Inappropriate, vigorous immune responses to foreign antigens, known as hypersensitivity reactions, can cause mild to severe damage to the host.

There are four classes of hypersensitivities, based on the underlying immune mechanism.

Many clinical hypersensitivity diseases have components of more than one class of hypersensitivity.

Hypersensitivity reactions usually require previous exposure to the inciting antigen and are rarely observed on primary exposure.

Acute Phase Response Infections and other inflammatory stimuli induce the rapid production of a group of proteins called acute phase proteins that enhance resistance to infection in a non–antigen-specific manner.

List of Principles — cont'd

The acute phase response prepares the body to eliminate or neutralize inflammatory stimuli and promotes tissue healing and repair.

The acute phase response has local and systemic components.

Neonatal Immunology

Newborn humans and animals receive antibodies from their mothers to help them ward off infectious diseases while their native defense mechanisms mature and as they develop active immune responses to the antigens they encounter.

Maternally derived antibodies may be obtained through the placenta or through colostrum in mammals and through the yolk sac in birds.

High titers of circulating maternal antibodies may prevent neonates from mounting their own immune responses to the antigens for which the antibodies are specific.

Milk contains antibodies that continue to provide local protection in the gastrointestinal tract.

No significant passive transfer of cell-mediated immunity occurs from mothers to neonates.

Immunology of Cancer

Cancer cells are cells that have undergone a change so that they multiply in an uncontrolled fashion. The immune system attacks and destroys most cancerous cells as they arise because it recognizes changes in the surface antigens of the cells.

Progressive cancers are characterized by cells that escape immune surveillance.

Immunotherapies for cancer seek to alter the surface antigens on cancer cells so that they are recognized and attacked by the immune system, or seek to activate immune cells to be more effective.

Immunose-nescence

The ability of the immune system to protect against infection and cancer and to avoid autoimmune disease decreases in advanced age.

The immune system in different individuals undergoes age-related changes (immunosenescence) at different rates and to different degrees.

Some cells and functions of the immune system are more affected by age than others.

TOPIC 1: Autoimmunity

Principles

1. An autoimmune state occurs when an individual's immune system ceases to tolerate certain self antigens and mounts an immune response to eliminate those antigens.
2. Autoimmunity may be generalized or organ specific.
3. Many factors contribute to the onset of autoimmune disease, including the genetic background of the affected individual and prior exposure to related antigens.

Explanation

The immune system must maintain a finely tuned balance between reactivity against any potential foreign antigens it may encounter and tolerance of those antigens normally found in the body (self antigens). Occasionally, an individual's immune system loses its tolerance for certain self antigens and begins to attack the individual's own tissues as if they were foreign invaders. This phenomenon is called *autoimmunity*. Several clinically recognized disease syndromes are due to underlying autoimmune processes, including multiple sclerosis, juvenile diabetes, Grave's disease, and systemic lupus erythematosus (SLE).

An autoimmune disease may be generalized, such as SLE, in which many different tissues and antigens are under immune attack. Others are organ specific, in which the immunological attack is restricted to one or a few self antigens. For example, the clinical effects of multiple sclerosis occur because of immunological destruction of the myelin sheaths on nerve fibers. Insulin-producing pancreatic cells are attacked in cases of juvenile diabetes, and thyroid cells are attacked in those with Grave's disease.

Generalized autoimmunity may occur from a defect in the ability of the immune system to generate or maintain self-tolerance, or it may occur from widespread, nonspecific immune activation, such as that associated with administration of superantigens or nonspecific lymphocyte stimulants (mitogens). Organ-specific autoimmunity, however, is probably better explained by an antigen-specific gap in tolerance, which might occur when the immune system is exposed to, and reacts against, a particular self antigen for which tolerance was never established.

Recognition of self antigens and establishment of tolerance to them occurs mainly during fetal life, but tolerance only is established toward antigens that are present in the local environment (thymus or bone marrow) of the developing lymphocytes. Some self antigens are specific for tissues in other parts of the body, so they may not be available in the thymus or bone marrow for recognition. Other complex self antigens, though present in the thymus or bone marrow, are arranged so that only certain reactive sites (epitopes) on their structure are presented to developing lymphocytes. Consequently, lymphocytes reactive against tissue-specific antigens or cryptic (hidden) epitopes may be released into circulation. In healthy individuals, however, these auto-reactive lymphocytes do not attack host tissues, perhaps because their complementary antigens/epitopes are buried deep within tissues and not readily exposed to the immune system or because they are never presented to the immune system along with the costimulatory signals necessary to activate an immune response.

Several theories have been proposed to explain why self antigens that are essentially ignored by the immune systems of healthy individuals become targets for attack in autoimmune individuals (Fig. 5-1). Many suggest that the primary event, or at least an aggravating factor, in the development of autoimmunity is microbial infection. The onset of, or exacerbation of, autoimmune diseases often occurs after an infection.

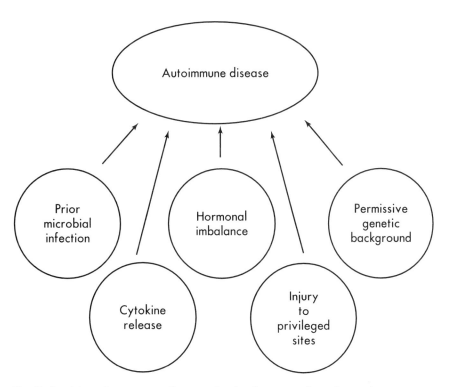

Fig. 5-1   Many factors contribute to the development of autoimmunity.

Even when there is no obvious history of infectious disease, it is possible that clinical recovery from the disease occurred long before clinical autoimmunity became apparent.

A microbial infection may cause tissue damage that exposes tissue-specific antigens or cryptic epitopes to the immune system. Antigens residing deep within the solid tissue of an organ may be relatively protected from exposure to the immune system because intact vascular walls and other anatomical barriers (e.g., blood-brain barrier) prevent easy migration of lymphocytes into the tissue. However, microbial infections can damage vascular walls and anatomical barriers so that lymphocytes pass freely into the tissue, where they may come into contact with these antigens.

Microbial infections also induce local inflammation within a tissue, which, among other things, serves to induce cytokine production by various cell types. Certain cytokines, particularly interferon-gamma, cause affected cells to alter the types and quantities of surface molecules that they express. Among the surface molecules that are affected are major histocompatibility complex (MHC) molecules and costimulatory molecules. Therefore, cells that cannot present antigens in a stimulatory manner to lymphocytes under normal conditions may, under inflammatory conditions, be able to present their antigens in a manner that elicits an immune response.

Molecular mimicry is another mechanism by which microbes can induce autoimmune responses. Certain bacterial or viral antigens resemble self antigens of mammals, and immune responses against these microbes can generate lymphocytes that subsequently attack self antigens. For example, the M protein of certain *Streptococcus* spp. is similar to myosin, a component of mammalian muscle. During a streptococcal infection, lymphocytes reactive against M protein are activated and induced to proliferate. After the infection is cleared, increased numbers of lymphocytes reactive against M protein persist in the host as a part of immunological memory. Because memory cells are more easily activated than naive lymphocytes, myosin may be antigenically similar enough to M protein to serve as a cross-reactive target for the M protein-specific memory lymphocytes, even though it would not have activated naive M protein-specific lymphocytes. Thus, molecular mimicry may explain why some patients suffer from autoimmune-mediated myocarditis (inflammation of the heart muscle) after streptococcal infections.

Neuroendocrine imbalances also have been identified as aggravating factors in the induction of autoimmunity. Most individuals suffering from autoimmune diseases are female, and onset often occurs near puberty or pregnancy, suggesting that sex hormones may play a role in initiating autoimmunity. It has been shown in animal models that alterations in corticosteroid, testosterone, estrogen, and prolactin production, as well as alterations in reactivity of the sympathetic nervous system, can enhance various types of autoimmunity.

Even though microbial infections and neuroendocrine imbalances have been implicated in the induction of autoimmunity, these events alone are not sufficient for the development of autoimmune disease. Autoimmune individuals also must possess a permissive genetic background. Immunologists have identified several groups of genes that may influence susceptibility to autoimmunity. It is unlikely that any individual gene determines susceptibility, and different genes are active in the development of different types of autoimmunity. Several autoimmunity-associated genes belong to histocompatibility gene clusters. This seems logical because MHC molecules play a critical role in how antigens are presented to lymphocytes. Antigen-presenting cells from individuals with a given type of MHC molecule might present certain foreign antigens so that they more closely resemble self antigens than might antigen-presenting cells from individuals with a different type of MHC molecule.

Immunologists are seeking to improve treatment options for individuals suffering from autoimmune disease. Currently most treatments involve the administration of antiinflammatory or cytotoxic drugs, such as corticosteroids or cyclophosphamide. The drawback of generalized immunosuppressive therapies is that while they retard autoimmune-mediated tissue destruction, they also suppress the ability of the immune system to respond to foreign antigens. Therefore, treatments that selectively suppress autoimmune activity without affecting immunity to other antigens are being sought.

Related Topics

T lymphocyte antigen recognition
Recognition of self vs. non-self
Tolerance
Memory lymphocytes

Additional Reading

Steinman, L. 1993. Autoimmune disease. Sci. Am. 269:106-114.
Theofilopoulos, A.N. 1995. The basis of autoimmunity: Part I. Mechanisms of aberrant self-recognition. Immunol. Today. 16:90-98.
Theofilopoulos, A.N. 1995. The basis of autoimmunity: Part II. Genetic predisposition. Immunol. Today. 16:150-159.

TERMS:

Autoimmunity   Condition in which the immune system attacks self antigens using humoral or cell-mediated immune mechanisms.

Cryptic Epitopes   Sites on an antigen that are not normally accessible to generate an immune response. Exposure of cryptic epitopes on self antigens to the immune system may induce autoimmunity.

Study Questions

1. What factors might precipitate the onset of autoimmunity?
2. How can microbial infection lead to autoimmune disease?
3. Why are immunologists seeking alternative treatment strategies to the conventional treatments for autoimmune diseases?

TOPIC 2: Transplantation

Principles

1. Transplanted tissues may be attacked and rejected by the immune system if the molecules on the cell surfaces of the transplanted tissue are antigenically different from those of the host.
2. Matching the MHC antigens of donor and recipient tissues before transplantation reduces the incidence of graft rejection.
3. Graft vs. host disease, in which the lymphocytes in the donor tissue attack the recipient, is a special type of transplantation reaction that may occur in severely immunocompromised individuals.

Explanation

Great advances have been made in the field of organ transplantation in recent years, but manipulating the recipient immune system to accept non-self tissue grafts remains one of the greatest challenges to successful transplantation. Transplanted tissues from any donor other than an identical twin possess antigens foreign to the recipient and thus have the potential to be attacked and destroyed (rejected) by the recipient immune system. Rejection can be minimized by matching antigens on donor and recipient tissues as closely as possible. Rejection responses based on minor tissue antigen mismatches then usually can be controlled or eliminated by suppressing the immune response of the recipient through drugs or antilymphocyte antibodies.

Practically any foreign antigen on transplanted tissues can serve as a target for immune rejection by the recipient, but the most important for tranplantation of organs between members of the same species are the major histocompatibility complex (MHC) molecules. Unlike other foreign antigens that must be presented to T lymphocytes in combination with self-MHC molecules to activate an immune response, allogeneic MHC molecules on the membranes of transplanted cells can stimulate recipient T lymphocytes directly; the mechanism by which this occurs is uncertain. Alternatively, allogeneic MHC molecules can stimulate recipient lymphocytes in the traditional manner. When MHC molecules are shed from transplanted cells, they may be internalized by recipient antigen-presenting cells, processed, and presented to recipient lymphocytes as peptides in combination with self-MHC molecules. For reasons that are yet unclear, the number of lymphocytes within an individual that are reactive against a given MHC allotype is 10 to 100 times greater than the number that are reactive against any other type of foreign antigen, so exposure to allogeneic MHC can elicit strong immune responses.

Graft rejection may be acute or chronic. Acute rejection may occur 1 to 2 weeks after transplantation. Subsequent transplants from the same donor may be rejected within 48 hours. This accelerated rejection is called a *second set reaction* and is due to immunological memory. Chronic rejection may occur at any time after transplantation and is highly variable in the time it takes to develop.

Rejection of transplanted tissues is mediated primarily by T lymphocytes. Both CD4+ and CD8+ lymphocytes are involved, but the relative contributions of each appear to depend on the type of tissue antigen incompatibility that exists between donor and recipient and the type of tissue being transplanted. Helper T lymphocytes recognizing differences in class II MHC may be involved in the initial recognition of foreign grafts by the recipient. Differences in class I MHC make the transplanted cells targets for cytotoxic T cell responses.

Cytotoxic antibodies directed against transplanted tissue also may be generated during a rejection episode. These antibodies probably play a role in the accelerated rejection of second set reactions. Class I and class II MHC alloantigens are both targets for antibody responses.

Recipient lymphocytes are first exposed to alloantigens when whole transplanted cells and/or antigens from the cells are shed from a graft and are transported in the lymph to local lymph nodes. There the alloantigens activate recipient lymphocytes, which proliferate and home to the graft. Activated lymphocytes accumulate in the graft, releasing toxic cytokines and participating in cellular cytotoxicity. The cytokines also attract nonspecific immune cells, such as macrophages, to the graft, which intensifies the inflammatory response. The resultant cellular damage to the graft, especially to the vasculature of the graft, causes the graft to undergo necrosis.

A special type of rejection response called *graft vs. host disease (GVHD)* may occur when bone marrow is transplanted. Bone marrow transplants contain large numbers of functional donor lymphocytes, and the recipient is immunosuppressed because the recipient's own bone marrow is obliterated in preparation for the transplant. Consequently, the donor lymphocytes, which recognize and are activated by the antigens they see as foreign in the recipient, begin to attack recipient tissues, whereas the recipient has little capacity to attack the donor cells. Cytokines released by the activated donor lymphocytes play a major role in the pathogenesis of GVHD because they amplify the effects of tissue damage that occurred while preparing the recipient for transplantation. The reaction, if not controlled, can be fatal to the recipient. Donor marrow can be depleted of mature T lymphocytes before transplantation to minimize the chances of developing GVHD, but this treatment also increases the chance of graft failure because T-cell depleted marrow may not restore full immunocompetence to the recipient.

Clinically, the profile of MHC molecules expressed by donor tissue is compared with that of potential recipients before transplantation in an effort to match donors with recipients possessing the most genetic similarities. The success rate for many types of tissue transplants (e.g., kidney, bone marrow) is greatly enhanced when MHC-matched tissues are used. Typically, serological tests are used to compare MHC molecules between donor and recipient, although other tests are available (Fig. 5-2). Several antisera, each prepared so that it is specific for a different allotype of MHC molecule, are mixed individually with samples of donor or recipient lymphocytes and complement. The lymphocytes will undergo complement-mediated lysis if they express the MHC allotype for which the antiserum is specific. Tissues are typed according to their pattern of reactivity with the various antisera. New methods that compare MHC allotypes at the genetic level, such as polymerase chain reaction and DNA restriction fragment analysis, are also being developed.

Tissues do not need to be genetically matched with the recipient before transplantation if no graft survival advantage is obtained by tissue matching. This most often occurs when the donor tissue is transplanted into an immune-privileged site, such as the cornea. Tissues transplanted into an immune-privileged site are tolerated by the recipient

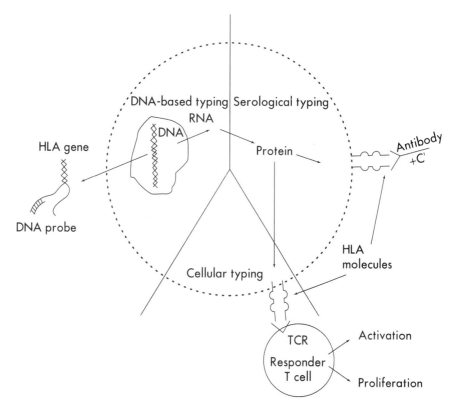

Fig. 5-2   Serological, cellular, and DNA typing approaches for MHC determination. Each of the MHC typing methods relies on detection of sequence variation—either nucleotide (DNA) or amino acid (protein) in the MHC molecules. DNA-based typing directly analyzes the DNA code after extraction of nucleic acids from any cell or tissue. Serological and cellular typing require the expression of the MHC molecules, usually on a lymphoid cell, and analyze the allogeneic determinants on the MHC protein, using antibodies or T-cell reactivity, respectively. (Modified from Rich, R.R. [ed.] 1996. Clinical Immunology: Principles and Practice. Mosby-Year Book, St. Louis.)

immune system, either because they are relatively sequestered from exposure to recipient lymphocytes (the cornea is usually avascular and has poor lymphatic drainage) or because they reside within an immunosuppressive local environment. A fetus is also a type of unmatched graft because it expresses paternal antigens that are foreign to the mother. The relative isolation of the placenta and fetus within the uterus and the locally immunosuppressive environment of the placental-uterine junction protect the fetus from attack by the maternal immune system.

Immunosuppressive therapies are often used in recipient individuals to prevent rejection of transplanted tissues from minor antigen mismatches. The most common drugs that are used in posttransplant immunosuppression are glucocorticoids (prednisone) and cyclosporin A, which suppresses production of interleukin-2 by activated lymphocytes. Sometimes these drugs require lifelong administration. In other cases, the use of immunosuppressive drugs can be reduced or eliminated after the threat of acute rejection has passed because peripheral tolerance for donor antigens may eventually develop in the recipient. The continual presence of the donor antigens may stimulate the production of lymphocytes with suppressor activity or cause reactive lymphocytes to become anergic.

Currently, the immunosuppressive therapies that are used clinically serve to suppress the recipient immune system in a nonspecific manner. It would be preferable to develop therapies that target donor-reactive lymphocytes specifically, leaving the rest of the recipient immune system to function normally. Experimental research on such strategies is under way, the approaches often overlapping with those being developed to treat autoimmunity.

Although allogeneic grafts are the type of transplant currently in clinical use, the feasibility of transplantation between animal species is being investigated. The use of domestic animals, such as the pig, as organ donors for humans would greatly reduce or eliminate chronic donor organ shortages. Transplants between animal species are called *xenografts*. Transplants between closely related species, such as apes and humans, are called *concordant xenografts;* grafts between evolutionarily distant species are called *discordant xenografts*.

Currently, discordant xenografts are rejected within minutes of transplantation by a complement-mediated mechanism. Xenografts quickly activate complement via the alternative pathway or the classical pathway, depending on whether the recipient possesses naturally occurring antibodies to the donor tissue. (Humans possess antibodies to pig tissues even though they have not been exposed previously to pig antigens.) Accumulation of complement complexes on the endothelial cells of the vasculature of the transplanted organ causes the formation of blood clots that occlude the blood vessels, destroying the integrity of the organ. This rapid, fulminant rejection process must be controlled before xenotransplantation can become a viable clinical alternative to allotransplantation. Researchers are currently attempting to produce genetically engineered pigs that have either pig-specific molecules removed from their cell surfaces or human-specific molecules added to their cell surfaces (or both) for use as organ donors.

Related Topics

Tolerance
Autoimmunity

Additional Reading

Ferrara, J.L.M. 1993. Cytokine dysregulation as a mechanism of graft vs. host disease. Curr. Opin. Immunol. 5:794-799.
Hutchinson, I. 1996. Transplantation and rejection. In Roitt, I., Brostoff, J., and Male, D. (eds.) Immunology. Mosby-Year Book, St. Louis.
Lu, C., Khair-El-Din, T., Davidson, I., Butler, T., Brasky, K., Vazquez, M., and Sicher, S. 1994. Xenotransplantation. FASEB J. 8:1122-1130.
Stepkowski, S.M. 1994. Transplantation immunobiology. An update. Surg. Clin. North Am. 74:991-1013.

TERMS:

Allograft	Graft from a nonidentical twin donor of the same species.
Graft vs. Host Reaction	Rejection reaction in which the donor lymphocytes attack recipient tissues. Graft vs. host reactions usually occur when the recipient is severely immunosuppressed.
Necrosis	Tissue death.
Second Set Reaction	Accelerated rejection reaction that occurs when an individual receives a second graft of the same tissue type as a previously rejected graft.
Xenograft	Graft from a donor of a different species.

Study Questions

1. What immune mechanisms are responsible for graft rejection?
2. What is graft vs. host disease, and when is it most likely to occur?
3. What are xenografts?
4. What molecules on cell surfaces are almost always different between individuals of the same species and are usually responsible for graft rejection?

TOPIC 3: Psychoneuroimmunology

Principles

1. The immune system, the nervous system, and the endocrine system influence one another.
2. The nervous system may influence the immune system through direct innervation of lymphoid tissues or through the release of neurotransmitter molecules.
3. Stress affects the quality and magnitude of immune responses.
4. Several hormones are capable of influencing immune function.

Explanation

Until the past decade or so, immunological dogma held that the immune system was an isolated, closed system, receiving input from and regulated by only its own components and antigens. However, the immune system is not isolated, but rather it is intricately interrelated with other body systems, including the nervous and endocrine systems (Fig. 5-3). Together these systems form the basis of a rapid and flexible response system for the countless, dynamic physiological and environmental challenges that may affect an individual. The study of the relationship between the immune and neuroendocrine systems, called *neuroimmunology* or *psychoneuroimmunology*, is growing rapidly as it becomes increasingly apparent that knowledge of the interactions between these body systems is as important to an overall understanding of immunology as knowledge of interactions within the immune system itself.

Communication between the immune system and the neuroendocrine system is bidirectional. It has been suggested that the immune system serves as a sensory system for the nervous system, translating signals from stimuli that the nervous system cannot receive directly (e.g., bacteria, viruses, tumors). Likewise, the neuroendocrine system can relay immediate, up-to-date information regarding the overall physiological status of the individual to the immune system.

The nervous system communicates with the immune system by two methods: direct innervation of lymphoid tissues and release of neurotransmitter molecules. Primary and secondary lymphoid tissues are richly innervated with nerves of the sympathetic branch of the autonomic nervous system (i.e., nerves involved in "fight or flight" responses to physical and psychological stressors). Some of the nerve endings are in direct contact with surfaces of lymphocytes and macrophages residing within the tissues. Their contacts have features similar to nerve-nerve synapses (junctions), so certain immune cells may be able to receive and

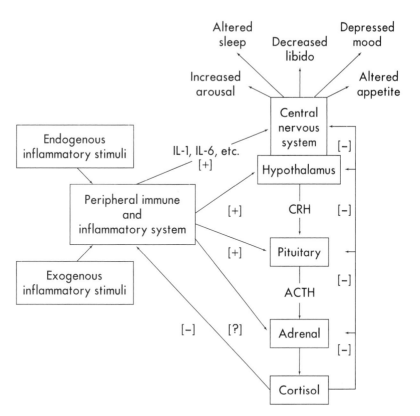

Fig. 5-3   The peripheral immune system, central nervous system, and hypothalamic-pituitary-adrenal axis (endocrine system) are integrated into a self-regulating feedback loop. CRH, corticotropin-releasing hormone; ACTH, adrenocorticotrophic hormone; IL, interleukin. (From Rich, R.R. [ed.] 1996. Clinical Immunology: Principles and Practice. Mosby-Year Book, St. Louis.)

interpret direct nerve impulses. Also, lymphocytes, macrophages, and neutrophils possess receptors for neurotransmitter molecules (norepinephrine) that are released during sympathetic nervous stimulation, making them responsive to changes in the nervous system even though they may not be in direct contact with nerve endings.

Many nerves within lymphoid tissues are associated with the blood vessels in the tissues. Nervous stimulation of the vasculature serves to alter local blood flow, thus affecting lymphocyte circulation through, and migration into, the tissue.

The immune system also receives input from the endocrine system, in the form of locally produced or circulating hormones. The hypothalamus and pituitary regions of the brain and the adrenal glands, also known as the *HPA axis,* are responsible for the production of many hormones with immunomodulatory properties (Table 5-1). Immune cells also are affected by gonadal hormones, such as testosterone and estrogen. Interestingly, immunologists are finding that immune cells not only contain receptors for many HPA axis-derived hormones but they also may produce analogues of many of the hormones themselves, making certain hormones mediators of bidirectional communication. Even though the

TABLE 5-1   SELECTED HORMONES WITH IMMUNOMODULATORY PROPERTIES*

Hormone	Effect on Immune Function
Adrenocorticotropin hormone (ACTH)	↓ Ab production; ↑ B cell proliferation; ↓ IFN-g production; ↓ MHC expression; ↑ NK cell activity
Corticosteriods	↓ circulating lymphocytes; ↓ IL-2, IL-1; ↓ MHC expression; ↓ lymphocyte migration
Corticotropin releasing hormone (CRH)	↑ IL-1, IL-6, TNF; ↑ NK cell activity
Growth hormone (GH)	↑ thymocyte proliferation; generally positive effect on immune function
Growth hormone releasing hormone (GHRH)	↑ lymph proliferation; ↓ NK cell activity
Prolactin	↑ differentiation of T cells; counters many suppressive effects of corticosteriods
Thyroid stimulating hormone (TSH)	↑ Ab production; ↑ B-lymphocyte differentiation
Luteinizing hormone (LH)	↑ lymphocyte proliferation; modulate Ab and cytokine production

*Receptors for these hormones have been identified on immune cells. Analogues of these hormones are produced by immune cells.

concentrations of leukocyte-derived hormones are much lower than those produced by the HPA axis, they may, nonetheless, play a significant role in the cross-regulation of the immune and neuroendocrine systems because of the ability of immune cells to circulate throughout the body and deposit hormones locally at their effector sites.

Immune cells also can communicate with the nervous and endocrine systems through the actions of cytokines. Interleukins-1, -2, -6, interferon-gamma, and tumor necrosis factor have been shown to affect the production of several HPA axis hormones. Interleukins-1 and -6 and tumor necrosis factor, through their acute phase effects, affect the nervous system and behavior by promoting sleep, decreasing appetite, and increasing the body temperature set point in the hypothalamus (fever). Cytokines, notably IL-1 and IL-6, are also produced locally by neurons and/or glial cells in several areas of the brain. The role of locally produced cytokines within the central nervous system is yet unclear, but they may serve to transmit communication signals provided by hormones and other molecules that are too large to cross the blood-brain barrier.

Numerous reports in the scientific literature describe specific effects of various hormones, neurotransmitters, or cytokines on specific immune or neuroendocrine functions, but the effect of a given cross-regulatory stimulus on an overall immune or neuroendocrine response probably depends on the timing and duration of the stimulus, the presence of other regulatory stimuli, and the nature of the underlying immune or neuroendocrine mechanism that is involved. This is particularly true of neurological influences on immune responses. Immune responses are generated over a course of days to weeks, whereas neural input tends to be instantaneous in its onset and of highly variable duration. Therefore, neural immunomodulation may have a different effect depending on, for example, whether it is applied at the time of initial antigenic recognition by naive B lymphocytes or after specific antibody production is well established. Duration is also important because it has been shown, for example, that acute physical exertion and chronic physical activity have opposite effects on the number of circulating lymphocytes.

Physical or psychological stress tends to depress immune function. This phenomenon has been demonstrated repeatedly, in studies linking stressful situations as diverse as college students during examination week or animals giving birth with depressed immune function and reduced resistance to illness. Corticosteroids, released by the adrenal glands during stressful episodes, mediate many, but not all, of the immunosuppressive effects seen during stressful periods. They may accomplish these effects through interference with cytokine production by immune cells.

Despite the general tendency for large doses of corticosteroids to suppress immune function, corticosteroids in smaller, physiological doses are essential for proper immune function. They play a role in the regulation of nearly every aspect of immune function and inflammation. Under normal circumstances, corticosteroids probably serve to control the magnitude of immune responses, protecting individuals from overreactivity.

Just as harmful stress tends to suppress immune function, inner peace and well-being have been implicated in enhancing immunity. The scientific basis for this effect appears to lie, in part, in the fact that lymphocytes, neutrophils, and platelets have receptors for opioid molecules, such as endorphins and enkephalins. Endorphins and enkephalins are molecules that reduce pain and produce a natural euphoria, but they also enhance cytotoxic T lymphocyte and natural killer cell activity and enhance cytokine production.

Immune responses can be conditioned in response to unrelated stimuli, much as Pavlov conditioned dogs to salivate whenever a bell was rung. For example, mice given a saccharin solution in combination with an immunsuppressive drug can eventually be conditioned so that they exhibit depressed immune parameters after receiving saccharin alone. Conditioned responses to elicit allergic reactions and to suppress delayed-type hypersensitivity reactions also have been reported. This phenomenon shows a link between behavior and immune function because the response is not always attributable to physical stress responses that might occur in response to receiving the initiating stimulus.

Even though the numerous links between brain, behavior, hormones, and immunity are interesting and can affect overall immune responses, it is important to remember that these cross-regulatory influences are not the primary regulators of immune function. There are no substitutes for the effects of direct antigenic challenge and functional immune cells. Conditioned reactions to unrelated stimuli cannot replace the need for efficacious vaccines, and a sense of well-being cannot overcome the effects of an immunodeficiency state. Cross-regulatory influences are but one factor in the complex physiological balance necessary for optimum immune function.

Related Topic

The acute phase response

Additional Reading

Husband, A.J. 1993. Role of the central nervous system and behaviour on the immune system. Vaccine. 11:805-816.

Khansari, D., Murgo, A.J., and Faith, R.E. 1990. Effects of stress on the immune system. Immunol. Today. 11:170-175.

Maier, S.F., Watkins, L.R., and Fleshner, M. 1994. Psychoneuroimmunology: the interface between behavior, brain, and immunity. Am. Psychol. 49:1004-1017.

Reichlin, S. 1993. Neuroendocrine-immune interactions. N. Engl. J. Med. 329:1246-1253.

Weigent, D.A. and Blalock, J.E. 1995. Associations between the neuroendocrine and immune systems. J. Leukoc. Biol. 57:137-150.

TERMS:

Hypothalamic-pituitary-adrenal (HPA) Axis	Communication feedback loop between the endocrine and nervous systems.
Neurotransmitter	Molecules used to transmit signals between nerve fibers.
Psychoneuro-immunology	The study of the interrelationships between the nervous system, immune system, and behavior.

Study Questions

1. Why is it advantageous for the immune, nervous, and endocrine systems to be linked?
2. How does the neuroendocrine system influence the immune system?
3. How does the immune system influence the neuroendocrine system?
4. How does stress suppress immunity?

TOPIC 4: Immunodeficiency

Principles

1. Many factors, including genetic defects, stress, viral infection, toxins, cancer, and old age can lead to defects in immune function.
2. Individuals with severe immunodeficiencies tend to have severe recurrent infections with unusual or opportunistic pathogens.
3. The characteristics of a recurrent infectious process may give clues as to the type of immunodeficiency by which an individual is affected.

Explanation

When any part of the immune system does not function properly, the ability to eliminate infectious agents and cancerous cells may become compromised. However, some aberrations in immune function are never apparent because the redundancy with which the immune system functions allows other cells and mechanisms to compensate for the defect. When the defect(s) in immune function are severe enough that an individual is at high risk for infections and/or cancers, that individual is said to be *immunodeficient.*

Immunodeficiencies may be primary or secondary. *Primary immunodeficiences* arise as the result of a hereditary or developmental defect in immune cells or cell function. *Secondary immunodeficiencies* arise as the result of an outside assault on the immune system, such as infections (e.g., HIV), immunosuppressive drugs, malnutrition, metabolic disease, cancer, or trauma. Most secondary immunodeficiencies are reversible if the primary insult can be corrected because there are no inherent defects in the immune system.

Immune defects may be quantitative or qualitative (i.e., there may be a reduction or absence of a particular type of immune cell or cell product, or there may be a functional defect that prevents effective immune responses despite normal or increased populations of cells.) Defects may occur in humoral immunity, cell-mediated immunity, or in native defense mechanisms. The defects also may occur in cells or molecules outside of the immune system but which affect the immune system, such as defects in major histocompatibility complex molecules. Table 5-2 contains a list of selected immunodeficiencies that have been described clinically in humans and animals.

Immunodeficient individuals tend to be most susceptible to a specific group of infectious agents, depending on what part of the immune response is impaired. For example, individuals with neutrophil defects often experience recurrent infections with extracellular bacteria, such as *Staphylococcus* spp., because neutrophils play a key role in the elimination of these pathogens. Depressed cellular immunity often leads to viral infections because cytotoxic T lymphocytes play a key role in the control of viruses.

The net state of immunosuppression that is experienced by immunodeficient individuals depends on a number of factors. The duration of the underlying defect is important because many immunodeficiencies develop over time. For example, individuals infected with the human immunodeficiency virus do not become clinically ill until a large proportion of their CD4+ lymphocytes have been destroyed directly or indirectly by the virus. Immunosuppressive drugs have variable effects depending on the timing of their administration; they may be less suppressive if given less frequently or in combination with other drugs. Concurrent diseases also may enhance the severity and progression of immunodeficiency states in affected individuals.

TABLE 5-2 SELECTED PRIMARY IMMUNODEFICIENCIES SEEN IN HU-MANS AND DOMESTIC ANIMALS

Name	Immune System Component Involved
Leukocyte adhesion deficiency	Integrin molecules
Chediak-Higashi syndrome	Neutrophil granules
Autosomal recessive severe combined immunodeficiency	T and B lymphocytes
Agammaglobulinemia	Antibody production
Selective IgA deficiency	B lymphocyte—class switching to IgA
C2 deficiency	Complement factor C2 (production or secretion)
Bare lymphocyte syndrome	MHC class II expression

Considerations for the diagnosis and medical management of immunodeficient individuals have received increased attention in recent years because of the AIDS epidemic. Immunodeficient individuals often are susceptible to clinical disease by pathogens that do not cause apparent infection in immunocompetent individuals; such pathogens are known as *opportunistic pathogens*. However, care must be taken in prescribing medical treatment for these individuals because they may experience additional side effects to commonly prescribed drugs. For instance, many orally administered antibiotics disrupt the normal intestinal flora, which is an important component of the native immune system. Without protective flora, pathogenic organisms may invade through the gut wall and cause disease that the immunodeficient individual cannot fight.

Diagnosis of disease is sometimes complicated in immunodeficient individuals. Although they are at increased risk for developing infections, immunodeficient individuals do not always show clinical symptoms of disease until the disease is well advanced. This is because immunodeficient individuals may not have normal inflammatory responses, and it is often the nonspecific signs of inflammation that first signal the presence of an infectious agent in the body. Immunologically based diagnostic tests for specific diseases, such as skin testing for delayed-type hypersensitivity against tuberculosis or measurement of antibody titers for exposure to toxoplasmosis, also may be of reduced value in the immunodeficient individual.

Vaccination of immunodeficient individuals may be of reduced value or even unsafe. The efficacy of vaccines depends on an adequate immune response after the introduction of an antigen, and immunodeficient individuals may not mount that response. Also, many vaccines contain attenuated live organisms, which although nonpathogenic in normal individuals, may cause disease in immunodeficient patients.

Immunologists are continually attempting to develop treatments to correct or to compensate for immunodeficiency states. The intravenous administration of antibodies has been evaluated as a treatment for antibody deficiencies. As immunologists learn more about the regulatory effects of cytokines, they may be able to develop treatments to enhance recovery from immunodeficient states after immunosuppressive drug therapy. By administering cytokines that enhance proliferation and function of lymphocytes, affected individuals may be able to rebuild adequate populations of lymphocytes in less time.

Additional Reading

Fischer, A. and Arnaiz-Villena, A. 1995. Immunodeficiencies of genetic origin. Immunol. Today 16:510-514.

Howard, R.J. 1994. Infections in the immunocompromised patient. Surg. Clin. North Am. 74:609-620.

Paul, M.E. and Shearer, W.T. 1996. Chapter 38. Approach to the evaluation of the immunodeficient patient. In Rich, R.R. (ed.) Clinical Immunology: Principles and Practice. Mosby-Year Book, St. Louis.

Rubin, R.H. and Ferraro, M.J. 1993. Understanding and diagnosing infectious complications in the immunocompromised host. Current issues and trends. Hematol. Oncol. Clin. North Am. 7:795-812.

TERMS:

Immunocompetent	Capable of mounting adequate and effective immune responses.
Primary Immunodeficiency	Immunodeficiency as a result of an inherited or congenital defect in the immune system.
Secondary Immunodeficiency	Immunodeficiency acquired as the result of disease, metabolic disturbances, malnutrition, or trauma.

Study Questions

1. Name three causes of secondary immunodeficiencies.
2. What type(s) of immunodeficiencies might predispose an individual to recurrent viral infections?
3. What types of immunodeficiencies might predispose an individual to recurrent bacterial infections?
4. What are opportunistic pathogens and what is the significance of diagnosing them as the cause of an infection?

TOPIC 5: Hypersensitivities

Principles

1. Inappropriate, vigorous immune responses to foreign antigens, known as hypersensitivity reactions, can cause mild to severe damage to the host.
2. There are four classes of hypersensitivities, based on the underlying immune mechanism.
3. Many clinical hypersensitivity diseases have components of more than one class of hypersensitivity.
4. Hypersensitivity reactions usually require previous exposure to the inciting antigen and are rarely observed on primary exposure.

Explanation

The immune system is a powerful defense mechanism against invasion by foreign antigens. However, many immune defenses, once they are deployed, have the potential to damage host tissues and the foreign antigens they are trying to eliminate. When immune responses are generated inappropriately or with undue strength in relation to the antigenic stimulus, the host may exhibit clinical signs of illness from the effects of the immune responses on healthy host tissues. These syndromes are called *hypersensitivities* (*hyper-* is the Latin root for "excess").

Individuals do not usually experience hypersensitivity reactions until they are exposed to an antigen for at least the second time. The naive animal on initial exposure to an antigen normally does not mount a strong enough response to cause detectable damage to host tissues. As discussed previously, lymphocytes capable of reacting against a certain antigen proliferate after the first exposure to that antigen, and B lymphocytes differentiate into plasma cells that can produce large quantities of specific classes of antibody. The second time that the host encounters an antigen, the immune response against that antigen is stronger and quicker. It is this strengthened immune response that causes the effect on the host to become pathological. Occasionally, if the initial dose of antigen is extremely large or if the antigen persists in the body, hypersensitivity reactions may occur on first exposure to antigen, but this is not usually the case.

There are four categories of hypersensitivity reactions, based on the types of immune cells or antibodies involved and the nature of the inciting antigen:

Type I hypersensitivity—immediate hypersensitivity

Type I, or immediate, hypersensitivity occurs within minutes of exposure to the inciting antigen. It is the type of response most closely associated with the lay term "allergic reaction." Localized type I hypersensitivity in the skin is commonly called *hives, wheals*, or *atopy*; in the upper respiratory tract, it is known as *hay fever*. If the hypersensitivity response is generalized and severe, it is called *anaphylaxis* (*ana-* meaning "opposite of" and *-phylax* meaning "protection").

Mediated by IgE antibodies, type I hypersensitivities are the result of mast cell and basophil degranulation. Mast cells are located in connective tissues and mucosal surfaces throughout the body, and basophils are present in circulation. IgE antibodies that have not yet bound to antigen can bind to receptors on the surface of mast cells and basophils. Binding of "empty" IgE molecules does not, in itself, affect these cells, but it readies them to mount a rapid response when antigen is encountered. When the appropriate antigens bind to mast cell- or basophil-associated IgE molecules (Fig. 5-4), signals are transmitted to the mast cell or basophil that induce the cells to release their cytoplasmic granules. The histamine and bradykinin in the granules mediate the undesirable effects associated with allergies and anaphylaxis.

Mast cell and basophil granules contain numerous molecules that increase vascular permeability, attract other inflammatory cells to the affected area, and function as anticoagulants or proteases. In addition to these preformed inflammatory factors, activation and degranulation of mast cells induce mast cells to produce additional substances that affect vascular tone and activate the complement and coagulation systems. All of these substances work together to produce the swelling, redness, and irritation we associate with allergies. If mast cell degranulation is widespread throughout the body (anaphylaxis), there is a rapid, massive shift in fluid balance from the vascular system to adjacent tissues, and the host goes into shock.

Systemic type I hypersensitivity (anaphylaxis) manifests itself clinically in different ways, depending on the host species. In humans and many domestic animals, the lung is the target organ, and affected individuals suffer respiratory distress. Dogs, cats, and horses also may

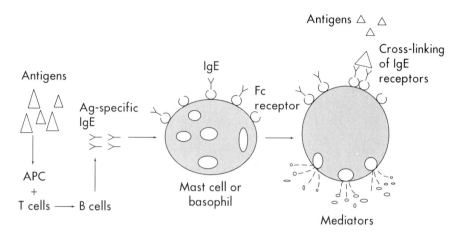

Fig. 5-4   Stages of IgE-mediated (type I) hypersensitivity reaction. Ag, antigen; APC, antigen-presenting cell; IgE, immunoglobulin E. (From Rich, R.R. [ed.] 1996. Clinical Immunology: Principles and Practice. Mosby-Year Book, St. Louis.)

have severe diarrhea during anaphylactic shock because the hepatic veins and/or intestine are shock organs in these species.

Type I hypersensitivities can be treated with epinephrine because it counteracts the effects of histamine and bradykinin. Steroids are useful for inhibiting the subsequent production of vasoactive substances by mast cells and basophils because they stabilize cellular membranes from which the inflammatory molecules are derived.

There appears to be a genetic predisposition for developing type I hypersensitivity reactions. In most individuals, IgE antibodies are present at very low levels, and they do not play a large enough role in immune responses to cause pathological reactions. Some individuals, however, have higher circulating levels of IgE and are more likely to experience hypersensitivities to various antigens.

Many individuals receive prophylactic treatment against type I hypersensitivities in the form of "allergy shots." The original theory behind this treatment, which is also called *hyposensitization,* was that by giving small, controlled doses of antigen in an alternative route to sensitized patients, production of IgG against the antigen would be stimulated. The elevated levels of IgG would be more likely to bind the inciting antigen before it could be bound by IgE. Immunologists now believe that the benefit of hyposensitization therapy lies in its ability to stimulate the production of interferon by macrophages. Interferon inhibits the differentiation and function of T_h2 lymphocytes, the lymphocyte subset that enhances the production of IgE, which may decrease IgE concentrations in circulation and in tissues.

Type II hypersensitivity—cytolytic hypersensitivity

Type II hypersensitivity is characterized by antibodies, primarily IgG, that attack cellular targets (Fig. 5-5). Normally, antibodies produced in the host are not directed against the host's own tissues; lymphocytes with self-antigen specificities are eliminated in the thymus. However, cells with surface antigens that the host recognizes as foreign are targets for attack by host antibodies. Such cells truly may be foreign, such as transfused blood cells, or they may be host cells that have atypical antigens on their surfaces because drugs or infectious agents have bound to them. In autoimmune diseases, the individual has a breakdown in tolerance and begins to make antibodies against its own red blood cells. When cells are bound by antibodies, they become marked for destruction. Circulating antibody-bound cells may be lysed by complement, and cells in extravascular locations may be ingested and destroyed by neutrophils and macrophages. Widespread destruction of a certain cell type can cause clinical disease.

The most common target cells for type II hypersensitivity reactions are red blood cells (RBCs). When many blood cells are destroyed at once, an individual becomes anemic because the bone marrow cannot produce enough RBCs to compensate for the loss. Also, the liver may not be able to process the breakdown products of the destroyed RBCs as quickly as they are generated, so the individual may become jaundiced. This is the pathological basis for blood transfusion reactions when blood from an incompatible donor group is given to previously sensitized recipients. It is also the pathogenesis for neonatal isoerythrolysis ("blue babies"). Moth-

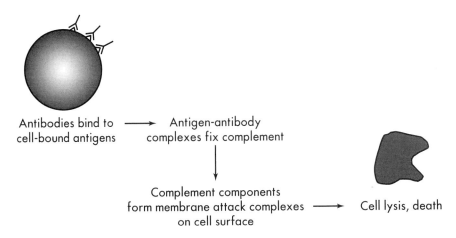

Antibodies bind to → Antigen-antibody
cell-bound antigens   complexes fix complement

Complement components
form membrane attack complexes → Cell lysis, death
on cell surface

Fig. 5-5   Type II hypersensitivity.

ers develop antibodies against paternally derived antigens during their first pregnancy. On subsequent pregnancies, these circulating antibodies attack paternally derived antigens on the baby's RBCs, causing massive hemolysis.

Drugs, such as penicillin, may bind to RBCs. Other drugs, such as sulfonamides, may bind to neutrophils or platelets. Type II hypersensitivities against these antigens may then result in anemia, neutropenia (usually manifested by recurrent bacterial infections), or clotting disorders.

Type III hypersensitivity—immune complex hypersensitivity

Type III hypersensitivity occurs when excess antigen-antibody complexes are formed in the host. It is similar to type II hypersensitivity in that it is mediated primarily by IgG, but instead of binding to cell-bound antigens, the antigens involved in type III hypersensitivity are soluble (Fig. 5-6). The antigen-antibody complexes can be relatively large, containing multiple molecules of both antigen and antibody. The complexes may adhere to endothelial cells in capillaries or accumulate in tissues. Like type II reactions, damage is mediated by complement and inflammatory cells (primarily neutrophils) that are attracted to the site of immune complex deposition. Type III hypersensitivity reactions take several hours after antigen exposure to develop; they reach maximal intensity in approximately 12 to 24 hours.

Obviously the binding of antibody to antigen is not, in itself, harmful to the host; it is the preliminary defense mechanism by which many

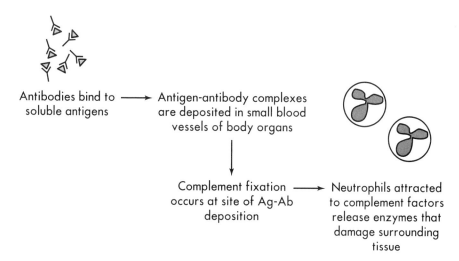

Antibodies bind to ⟶ Antigen-antibody complexes
soluble antigens   are deposited in small blood
    vessels of body organs

Complement fixation ⟶ Neutrophils attracted
occurs at site of Ag-Ab   to complement factors
deposition   release enzymes that
   damage surrounding
   tissue

Fig. 5-6 Type III hypersensitivity.

foreign antigens are removed from the body. The damage occurs when there are large numbers of antigen-antibody complexes that cannot be eliminated efficiently or when there is a chronic, continuous supply of complexes in a certain tissue. Hypersensitivity is most likely to develop when there is slightly more antigen than antibody because this ratio produces complexes that are the optimum size for deposition in blood vessel walls and tissues.

Antigen-antibody complexes trigger the classical pathway of complement activation, which produces inflammatory mediators that attract neutrophils and other inflammatory cells to the site. Neutrophils and macrophages contain many enzymes that can damage host tissues if they are "leaked" into the extracellular space, and substantial amounts of enzymes are released within the intense inflammatory foci that develop during type III reactions.

The classical example of localized type III hypersensitivity is the *Arthus reaction*, named after the scientist who first described it. Several hours after antigen is injected into the skin of a sensitized host, redness and swelling occur. If the inflammation is severe enough, the skin around the injection site will slough (necrosis). Microscopically, the site is characterized by the presense of many neutrophils and small clots (thrombi) in the small blood vessels.

Generalized type III hypersensitivity is called *serum sickness,* because it was first described when it was popular to administer antiserum as a treatment for diphtheria and tetanus. Sensitized individuals receiving large amounts of horse antiserum developed edema, arthritic pain, and vascular inflammation several days after treatment. These symptoms were caused by the large number of circulating antibody-antigen complexes (the antigen in this case being horse antibody molecules) that lodged in vascular walls and joints. The symptoms subsided as the complexes eventually were eliminated from circulation.

Type III hypersensitivity is a pathogenic component of many chronic infectious and autoimmune diseases. There are a number of infectious agents, including equine infectious anemia virus and aleutian mink disease virus, against which the host cannot generate neutralizing antibodies. The host produces large amounts of antibodies against these agents, but because they are not effective in eliminating the agent, the antibodies and antigen persist in the host indefinitely. The immune complexes are most likely to be deposited within the kidney, joints, and the walls of small blood vessels, causing persistent glomerulonephritis, arthritis, and vasculitis. Similarly, individuals suffering from autoimmune diseases produce antibodies against self antigens. If the self antigens against which the antibodies are directed are soluble, similar syndromes ensue.

Type IV hypersensitivity—cell-mediated hypersensitivity

Type IV hypersensitivity is mediated by T lymphocytes instead of antibodies. Because it takes a few days after exposure to antigen to develop in a sensitized individual, it is also called *delayed-type hypersensitivity (DTH)*. Type IV reactions occur when T lymphocytes are activated by antigen (Fig. 5-7). The cytokines produced by the antigen-specific lymphocytes attract other lymphocytes and macrophages and stimulate them to proliferate at the site of the reaction. Type IV reactions are not apparent until about 24 hours after antigen exposure, and it may take several days for the reaction to peak. It may take several weeks to months for DTH lesions to resolve completely, assuming that the antigen was eliminated. DTH lesions in the presence of chronic antigens may persist for years.

The most common example of type IV hypersensitivity is the tuberculin reaction. Individuals who have been previously exposed to tuberculosis-causing *Mycobacterium* spp. develop a hard swelling 24 to 96 hours after intradermal injection with mycobacterial extracts. This reaction is used as a diagnostic screening test for tuberculosis in humans and animals.

Contact hypersensitivity is also an example of delayed hypersensitivity. It occurs when T lymphocytes are activated by an antigen on the skin, and a red, pruritic (itchy) lesion develops many hours later. Sometimes the substances that elicit contact hypersensitivity are very small and would not elicit an immune response by themselves, but they become antigenic when they bind with proteins in the skin. Reactions to poison

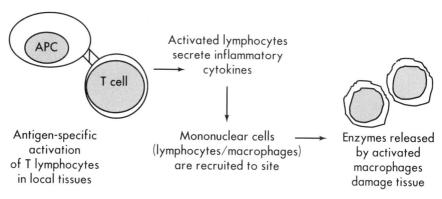

Fig. 5-7   Type IV hypersensitivity.

ivy fall into this category, as do allergic reactions against many chemicals. Clinically, contact hypersensitivity reactions in the skin may resemble immediate hypersensitivity reactions, but the time of onset is different. Also, type IV reactions are not characterized by high levels of IgE but rather by accumulations of lymphocytes and other mononuclear cells. Contact hypersensitivities do not respond well to hyposensitization therapy.

Most hypersensitivity reactions in vivo are probably a combination of one or more types. Many autoimmune diseases have features of both type II and type III reactions, especially if the antigen-antibody complexes bind to cells. Some allergies may involve type I and type IV components; immunologists now believe that flea allergies in cats and dogs represent a mixed type I and type IV reaction.

It is important to remember that the basic immunological reactions involved in hypersensitivities are not inherently pathological. For example, the mechanisms described for type I hypersensitivities—binding of antigen by IgE and degranulation of mast cells—are often used beneficially by the host to eliminate parasites. Also, accumulations of mononuclear cells, which are characteristic of type IV reactions, can be helpful to wall off pathogens from surrounding tissues and prevent their spread within the host. It is the magnitude of these responses or the locations at which these responses occur that makes hypersensitivity reactions damaging to the host.

Related Topic

Autoimmunity

Additional Reading

Strober, W. (ed.) 1996. Section 5: Allergic diseases. In Rich, R.R. (ed.) Clinical Immunology: Principles and Practice. Mosby-Year Book, St. Louis.

Tizard, I. 1996. Chapter 26. Type I hypersensitivity. In Veterinary Immunology: An Introduction, 5th ed. W.B. Saunders, Philadelphia.

Tizard, I. 1996. Chapter 27. Red cell antigens and type II hypersensitivity. In Veterinary Immunology: An Introduction, 5th ed. W.B. Saunders, Philadelphia.

Tizard, I. 1996. Chapter 28. Immune complexes and type III hypersensitivity. In Veterinary Immunology: An Introduction, 5th ed. W.B. Saunders, Philadelphia.

Tizard, I. 1996. Chapter 29. Type IV hypersensitivity: delayed hypersensitivity. In Veterinary Immunology: An Introduction, 5th ed. W.B. Saunders, Philadelphia.

TERMS:

Anaphylaxis	Shock reaction secondary to type I hypersensitivity reaction.
Atopy	A form of type I hypersensitivity.
Class I Hypersensitivity	Also known as immediate hypersensitivity because it occurs within minutes of exposure to antigen; characterized by mast cell and basophil degranulation subsequent to binding of IgE to antigen.
Class II Hypersensitivity	Cytolytic hypersensitivity caused by antibodies binding to nonsoluble antigen (usually cell-bound). The antigen-antibody complexes activate complement, leading to cell lysis by the membrane attack complex of complement.
Class III Hypersensitivity	Immune complex hypersensitivity caused by antibodies that bind to soluble antigen. The antigen-antibody complexes are deposited in small vessels of various body organs, and neutrophils and other inflammatory factors that are recruited to the site of antigen deposition mediate tissue damage.
Class IV Hypersensitivity	Also called delayed hypersensitivity because its onset is 24 to 48 hours after exposure to antigen. Characterized by mononuclear cell (T lymphocytes and monocytes/macrophages) accumulation at the site of antigen deposition.
Hyposensitization	Method of preventing or ameliorating type I hypersensitivities. The affected individual receives increasing doses of the inciting antigen through an alternative route that stimulates IgG, instead of IgE, production against the antigen.

Study Questions

1. What immune cell or molecule is the chief mediator of each type of hypersensitivity?
2. Why do hypersensitivities rarely occur on first exposure to an antigen?
3. What is the difference between type II and type III hypersensitivity? What are the similarities?
4. What is the mechanism by which hyposensitization therapy may help reduce the symptoms of type I hypersensitivity?

TOPIC 6: Acute Phase Response

Principles

1. Infections and other inflammatory stimuli induce the rapid production of a group of proteins called acute phase proteins that enhance resistance to infection in a non–antigen-specific manner.
2. The acute phase response prepares the body to eliminate or neutralize inflammatory stimuli and promotes tissue healing and repair.
3. The acute phase response has local and systemic components.

Explanation

In health, the organ systems of the body exist in an equilibrium (homeostasis). Whenever that equilibrium is altered by infection, injury, neoplasia (cancer), or other tissue damage, the body seeks to regain homeostasis. The body's response to such changes is called *inflammation,* and the inflammatory processes that occur immediately after detection of the inciting stimulus are collectively called the *acute phase reaction.*

The acute phase reaction has been described in humans and numerous species of animals, including some invertebrate species. The specific molecules that mediate the acute phase reaction may vary among species, but the overall objective of the process is essentially the same. The acute phase reaction is a complex, dynamic process that prepares the body to eliminate or neutralize the inflammatory stimulus and promotes tissue healing and repair. Even though the effects of the acute phase reaction are manifest mainly by clinical alterations in the immune, cardiovascular, and central nervous systems, all major systems of the body are involved.

Regardless of the nature of the inciting stimulus, the effects of the subsequent acute phase reaction are similar. The reaction is not antigen specific and utilizes native immune defenses. However, some infectious agents are more efficient than others at inducing an acute phase reaction. For example, bacterial infections often induce stronger reactions than viral infections, but this may be related more to the amount of tissue damage that a given infectious agent causes in the host than to any inherent properties of the infectious agent itself.

The acute phase reaction may be divided into local and systemic phases (Fig. 5-8). The local phase involves the initial changes that occur at the site of injury or infection. Cells that are activated locally release molecular mediators into the circulation that effect systemic changes throughout the body.

Local changes are mediated primarily through tissue macrophages or blood monocytes. Many bacterial products can activate macrophages

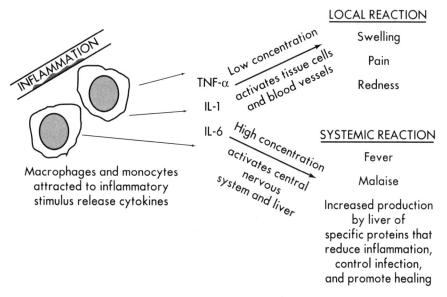

Fig. 5-8   The acute phase response.

directly. Mast cell degranulation, which may occur in response to parasitic infection or allergic reactions, causes the release of molecules that activate eosinophils and macrophages and attracts them to sites of inflammation. Alternatively, tissue damage in the absence of infection can also activate macrophages and monocytes through factors that are produced when platelets adhere to damaged blood vessels or cellular enzymes escape from damaged cells.

Macrophages, once they have been activated by an inflammatory stimulus, quickly produce several cytokines, many of which may participate to some extent in the acute phase response, but the most important are interleukin-1 (IL-1) and tumor necrosis factor (TNF). Macrophage-derived IL-1 and TNF, sometimes called *alarm cytokines,* act locally to activate connective tissue cells (fibroblasts) within inflamed tissues and endothelial cells of adjacent blood vessel walls. These activated cells produce additional cytokines and factors that cause blood vessels to dilate and become more permeable. They also stimulate the migration of additional leukocytes into the area of inflammation. The recruited leukocytes are, in turn, activated and secrete additional cytokines. The net result of this local cascade of cytokines is edema (swelling), pain, and redness.

As more cells become involved in producing cytokines in response to the inflammatory stimulus, the concentrations of cytokines in the circulation are elevated enough that they can mediate systemic changes. Among these systemic changes are an increase in body temperature and a general sense of illness, or malaise. Interleukins-1 and -6 and TNF have been implicated as mediators of the febrile response, which is achieved by altering the "set point" of the hypothalamus, the area of the brain that regulates body temperature. Fever and malaise are considered protective mechanisms during an inflammatory episode. An increase in body temperature causes a corresponding increase in the metabolic rate of the individual, which may serve to hasten the processes leading to the elimination of inflammatory stimuli. Also, certain infectious agents are less able to survive and multiply in a febrile host. Malaise serves to keep an individual quiet, which helps to keep the individual from mingling with others and spreading disease, and which allows the individual's energies to be focused on containing and resolving the focus of inflammation.

One of the major systemic effects of the acute phase reaction is an alteration in the types and quantities of proteins produced by the liver. Cytokines IL-1, IL-6, and TNF alter the pattern of protein production in liver cells by inducing specific protein-encoding genes to be more active. Proteins that are produced at a greater rate during an acute phase response are called *acute phase proteins* or *acute phase reactants*. Within 24 hours, their production may increase two to fiftyfold. The concentration of a few major acute phase reactants may be increased up to 1000-fold. The production of other proteins, called *negative acute phase proteins,* decreases to allow the liver to focus on the production of acute phase reactants.

Several types of proteins are considered acute phase reactants, including complement components, proteinase inhibitors, coagulation proteins, and metal-binding proteins. The complement system helps to resolve inflammation by acting as an opsonin to enhance clearance of inflammatory debris, recruiting inflammatory cells to sites of inflammation, and by lysing certain cells, such as gram negative bacteria, through the molecular attack complex. Proteinase inhibitors neutralize tissue-destroying enzymes (proteinases) that leak from damaged cells, thus limiting the spread of inflammatory-induced tissue damage to adjacent cells. Coagulation proteins serve to organize fibrin clots in damaged blood vessels, limiting the leakage of blood into underlying tissues. Certain metal-binding proteins bind to iron so that the host's iron supply cannot be utilized as a nutrient by bacteria. They also can act as scavengers for oxygen radicals, which are unstable molecules produced by activated inflammatory cells that can mediate tissue damage.

The three most abundant acute phase proteins are serum amyloid A, C-reactive protein, and serum amyloid P component. Ironically, less is understood about the functions of these proteins than some of the other minor acute phase reactants, but immunologists believe that they also serve to contain and resolve inflammation. Serum amyloid A inhibits oxygen radical production by neutrophils and inhibits IL-1 and TNF-induced fever. C-reactive protein and serum amyloid P component can activate complement, act as opsonins to enhance phagocytosis, and bind to nuclear chromatin, which aids in the uptake of damaged tissue cells by neutrophils and macrophages.

Serum levels of acute phase proteins may be measured to monitor the severity and the resolution of inflammation. The serum concentration of C-reactive protein is roughly proportional to the severity of an inflammatory process, and physicians monitor decreases in C-reactive protein levels to determine if internal inflammatory processes are resolving.

The acute phase reaction usually lasts only about 24 to 48 hours before it begins to subside. Background levels of acute phase reactants are often reestablished within 72 hours. The cytokines that mediate the acute phase reaction have a short half-life, so if the inflammatory stimulus is neutralized or eliminated, the level of circulating cytokines quickly diminishes. Also, many of the cytokines ultimately participate in regulatory feedback loops that limit the magnitude of their inflammatory effects. However, if the inflammatory stimulus is not neutralized or eliminated, the inflammatory process may enter a chronic phase. Little is known about the conditions that cause inflammation to convert from an acute to a chronic phase.

Chronic high-level production of acute phase reactants may be damaging to the host. Growth rates will decline and a decrease in muscle mass may occur. Serum amyloid proteins then begin to be deposited within various organs, a condition called *secondary* or *reactive amyloidosis*. Amyloid deposits within the spleen, kidney, and liver may lead to organ dysfunction. Reactive amyloidosis is commonly observed in chronic inflammatory diseases such as systemic lupus erythematosus and rheumatoid arthritis.

Related Topic

The complement system

Additional Reading

Baumann, H. and Gauldie, J. 1994. The acute phase response. Immunol. Today. 15:74-80.
Kushner, I. 1993. Regulation of the acute phase response by cytokines. Perspect. Biol. Med. 36:611-622.

Steel, D.M. and Whitehead, A.S. 1994. The major acute phase reactants: C-reactive protein, serum amyloid P component and serum amyloid A protein. Immunol. Today, 15:81-88.

TERMS:

Acute Phase Proteins	Proteins, mainly produced by the liver, that are produced in increased quantities during the acute phase response. Include complement components, proteinase inhibitors, coagulation proteins, and metal-binding proteins and other proteins with ill-defined functions.
Acute Phase Reaction	Collective term for local and systemic responses to inflammation. The acute phase response prepares the body to eliminate or neutralize inflammatory stimuli and prepares the body for healing. It occurs immediately after inflammation is detected and usually resolves within 24 to 48 hours.

Study Questions

1. Name three major classes of acute phase proteins.
2. What clinical signs may be seen during an acute phase response?
3. How does the acute phase reaction help an individual to fight infections?
4. What is the normal time course of the acute phase response?
5. How does the acute phase reaction affect an individual if it persists for a long time?

TOPIC 7: Neonatal Immunology

Principles

1. Newborn humans and animals receive antibodies from their mothers to help them ward off infectious diseases while their native defense mechanisms mature and as they develop active immune responses to the antigens they encounter.
2. Maternally derived antibodies may be obtained through the placenta or through colostrum in mammals and through the yolk sac in birds.
3. High titers of circulating maternal antibodies may prevent neonates from mounting their own immune responses to the antigens for which the antibodies are specific.

4. Milk contains antibodies that continue to provide local protection in the gastrointestinal tract.
5. No significant passive transfer of cell-mediated immunity occurs from mothers to neonates.

Explanation

Neonatal humans and animals are particularly susceptible to infectious diseases because their immature immune systems cannot yet eliminate invading pathogens efficiently and rapidly. To improve their immune defenses during the perinatal period, neonates receive passive immunity from their mothers. Mammals receive maternal antibodies via the placenta before birth or through the ingestion of colostrum immediately after birth.

Native immune responses are suboptimal during the perinatal period. Hence, neonates are particularly susceptible to infectious diseases caused by agents that may not cause disease in older animals. Phagocytosis is compromised because it takes several months, depending on the host species and type of cell, for phagocytic cells (i.e., neutrophils, macrophages) to function at adult levels. It also takes time to establish protective microbial flora on mucosal surfaces. Because the uterus provides a highly protected, and usually sterile, environment for developing fetuses, animals and humans are usually born with sterile mucosal surfaces. They are exposed to environmental microbes immediately after birth, but this flora must establish itself as a stable population on the various mucosae before it can begin to provide a defensive barrier against invading pathogens.

Antigen-specific immunity is also sluggish during the perinatal period. Lymph nodes develop relatively late in gestation, and unless the fetus experiences an infection against which it mounts an immune response while in the uterus, the lymph nodes are still somewhat underdeveloped at birth. The lymphocytes within neonatal lymph nodes are largely virgin cells that have never encountered their complementary antigen. Therefore, neonates mount primary immune responses, which can take 1 to 2 weeks to develop, against pathogens they encounter within the first hours and days of life. The lag time between exposure to the pathogen and onset of protective immunity may be long enough to allow serious disease to develop in the individual.

Mammals are not able to mount efficient immune responses against all types of antigens immediately after birth. Although neonatal lymphocytes can recognize and be activated by proteinaceous antigens even before birth, lymphocyte responses to carbohydrate antigens may be minimal until the immune system has matured. Humans do not respond efficiently to carbohydrate antigens until they are approximately 2 years old. This nonresponsiveness to carbohydrate antigens becomes clinically important when attempting to vaccinate young individuals against certain diseases. For example, *Neisseria meningitidis*, an organism that can cause fatal meningitis in young children, has a carbohydrate capsule that protects it from phagocytosis by immune cells. Effective vaccines have been developed that are aimed at generating opsonizing antibodies against the capsule so that the organism can more easily be phagocytosed and destroyed, but children younger than 2 years old do not respond well to vaccines containing capsular antigens.

Maternal antibodies provide an effective means of passive immunity to certain common pathogens to protect neonates until they can generate their own immune responses to these antigens. Neonates obtain a variable amount of maternal antibody before birth through transfer of immunoglobulins across the placenta. The amount of antibody that can be obtained transplacentally depends on the number of cell layers between the maternal and fetal vasculature. Primates and rodents receive most maternal antibodies, approximately 90%, via the placenta; immunoglobulins pass easily across the placenta because these species have only three placental cell layers between maternal blood and fetal blood. Dogs and cats, which have an additional placental cell layer, receive only 5% to 10% of maternal antibodies in utero. Domestic livestock (e.g., cattle, sheep, pigs, horses) do not receive maternal antibodies across the placenta. Their placentae, which are composed of five or six cell layers, are too thick to allow transfer of immunoglobulin molecules between mother and fetus.

Immunoglobulins received transplacentally are mainly of the IgG isotype. IgM antibodies are too large to cross vascular walls, and the remaining isotypes are present in maternal blood in such small quantities that transfer of these isotypes is negligible.

Birds also receive maternal antibodies before birth. Maternal antibodies are transfered to the egg yolk while it is still on the ovary. Chicks subsequently absorb yolk antibodies into their own circulation. Chicks obtain local antibodies for intestinal protection when they swallow egg-white fluid, which also contains maternal antibodies.

Colostrum provides another important means for the transfer of immunity between mother and offspring in mammals. Colostrum is the specialized mammary secretion that is produced immediately after birth, and it is rich in immunoglobulins. Colostral immunoglobulins are produced locally by the mammary gland, but a variable proportion is also derived from serum. IgG antibodies are the predominant isotype in the colostrum of most species, except for primates, where IgA predominates. However, significant quantities of IgA, which is the most important isotype for providing local immunity on mucosal surfaces, are present in colostrum of all species. Colostrum also contains maternal lymphocytes, but cell-mediated immunity does not appear to be passively transfered to neonates through colostral lymphocytes. Therefore, neonates do not receive passive immunity to diseases that require cell-mediated immune mechanisms for protection.

Colostrum is especially critical for those species of animals that receive little or no maternal antibody via the placenta. It is important for the neonate to ingest sufficient quantities of colostrum within the first few hours of life because it is during this time that the intestinal tract of the neonate is able to absorb large immunoglobulin proteins intact. After 6 to 12 hours, the intestinal tract begins to lose its permeability for large molecules and starts producing enzymes that degrade large dietary proteins before they are absorbed. By 24 hours, the intestine is unable to absorb ingested immunoglobulins. However, the neonate can still benefit from the local immunoglobulin activity of milk-derived secretory IgA molecules within the intestine, which serve to neutralize microbial toxins within the gut and prevent attachment of certain microbes to the gut wall. This local protective effect of milk-derived IgA will last as long as the neonate continues to receive milk from its mother.

Although maternally derived antibodies are critical for enhancing immune defenses in neonates, the presence of maternal antibodies can interfere with the production of active immune responses by young individuals. If the individual encounters an antigen that the circulating maternal antibodies recognize, the maternal antibodies can effectively inhibit response to that antigen by the host. They may do this by binding to that antigen so that it is quickly eliminated before it interacts with host lymphocytes (antigen sequestration), or they may cover the antigens when they bind to them so that they become unrecognizable by lymphocytes that have receptors for that antigen (antigen masking). In addition, maternal antibodies and other nonimmunoglobulin factors in colostrum mediate a transient, centralized suppression of the host immune system.

The effects of maternal antibody-mediated immunosuppression subside as maternal antibodies are degraded and are eliminated from circulation. Eventually the concentration of circulating maternal antibodies becomes so low that it is no longer immunosuppressive, and the young individual is able to mount its own immune response against a particular antigen. The length of time that maternal antibodies interfere with active immune responses depends on the original amount of antibodies that were received from the mother and their rate of degradation (half-life) in circulation. The half-life of IgG antibody molecules in most mammalian species is about 21 days.

The effect of immune interference by maternal antibodies is clinically important because the minimum antibody titer that protects an individual from a specific disease is often higher than the titer at which an individual can mount its own active immune response against that disease pathogen (Fig. 5-9). Consequently, when an individual has a maternal antibody titer that lies between these two points, it is susceptible to disease but unresponsive to vaccines containing that pathogen. Also, protective titers are not defined for many pathogens nor are titers at which maternal interference is no longer clinically significant, so this critical period of susceptibility is often ill-defined.

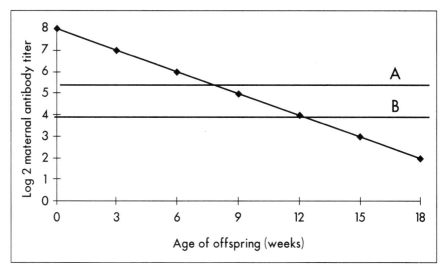

Fig. 5-9   Maternal antibodies to a given infectious agent, acquired through colostrum and/or the placenta, are eliminated from circulation at a constant rate during neonatal life. At some point (**A**), the maternal antibody titer becomes low enough that it is no longer sufficient to protect against disease in the neonatal animal. However, the titer at which the presence of maternal antibodies no longer suppresses an active immune response against that infectious agent by the neonate is often lower (**B**). In the time interval between A and B, the individual is susceptible to disease caused by the infectious agent but is not responsive to vaccination against that agent.

Additional Reading

English, B.K. 1996. Chapter 48. The neonatal immune response. In Rich, R.R. (ed.) Clinical Immunology: Principles and Practice. Mosby-Year Book, St. Louis.

Tizard, I. 1996. Chapter 19. Immunity in the fetus and newborn. In Veterinary Immunology: An Introduction, 5th ed. W.B. Saunders, Philadelphia.

TERMS:

Antigen Masking	Circulating antibodies bind to antigen, thus covering up essential epitopes on the antigen so that they cannot be recognized by lymphocytes.
Antigen Sequestration	Circulating antibodies bind to free antigen so that it is not available for processing by antigen-presenting cells for presentation to lymphocytes.
Colostrum	Specialized mammary secretion containing high levels of antibodies that is available to the newborn immediately after birth. Ingestion of adequate amounts of colostrum is essential to neonatal immunity in many animal species.
Immune Interference by Maternal Antibodies	Phenomenon whereby the presence of maternally derived antibodies to a specific infectious agent in the circulation of the newborn prevents the newborn from mounting a vigorous active immune response against that agent.

Study Questions

1. How do maternally derived antibodies interfere with the generation of active immune responses by neonates?
2. Why is the ingestion of colostrum critical for adequate immunity in some species more than in others?
3. In what ways are neonates immunodeficient?
4. How does continued ingestion of milk from the mother benefit the neonate?

TOPIC 8: Immunology of Cancer

Principles

1. Cancer cells are cells that have undergone a change so that they multiply in an uncontrolled fashion. The immune system attacks and destroys most cancerous cells as they arise because it recognizes changes in the surface antigens of the cells.

2. Progressive cancers are characterized by cells that escape immune surveillance.
3. Immunotherapies for cancer seek to alter the surface antigens on cancer cells so that they are recognized and attacked by the immune system, or seek to activate immune cells to be more effective.

Explanation

Normal cells in the body are subject to strict regulatory controls on their ability to proliferate and differentiate. These controls are necessary to maintain homeostasis among all body systems. However, replicating cells are constantly subject to genetic errors (mutations) that may affect how they respond to regulatory controls. Mutated cells are routinely generated throughout the life of an individual, but they are usually recognized by the immune system as abnormal cells and eliminated. Occasionally, mutated cells are not recognized as foreign by the immune system. If the mutation(s) within tolerated cells are located in genes that render the cells unresponsive to proliferative controls, uncontrolled cell division occurs and tumors develop.

Immunologists have long been interested in how cancerous cells escape immune detection and elimination. They also have searched for ways to manipulate tumors and/or the immune system so that immune responses can be generated against tumors as a method of cancer therapy. Great advances in tumor immunology have been made within the past decade, and many promising immunotherapies are being investigated.

A cancer cell might not be recognized as foreign by the immune system for several reasons. It may not express any antigens that differ from normal host cells, antigens from cancer cells may not be presented efficiently to potentially reactive lymphocytes, or lymphocytes may not be stimulated to generate an immune response after recognizing cancer cell antigens.

Cancerous tumors assume an altered appearance (morphology) from normal cells, so it is likely that they express different antigens from normal cells. However, these antigens are not always foreign antigens. Many cancer-associated antigens are developmental antigens, which are produced by normal host genes but limited in normal cells to expression only during fetal development. Their expression on mature cells is abnormal, but they are not inherently foreign, so the immune system does not mount an immune response against them.

Other cancerous cells do express antigens that are unique and thus foreign to the host's immune system. Immune nonresponsiveness to tumor-associated foreign antigens probably occurs because of improper antigen presentation or ineffective lymphocyte stimulation. Many tumors express low levels of major histocompatibility complex (MHC) molecules, which are necessary for antigen presentation to T lymphocytes. T lymphocytes cannot recognize antigens and be activated unless the antigens are presented in conjunction with MHC molecules. Tumors also rarely express costimulatory molecules (e.g., B7) that are necessary to activate lymphocytes once they have recognized their complementary antigen. Antigen recognition in the absence of costimulatory signals may induce anergy in T lymphocytes, rendering them unresponsive to subsequent contacts with their complementary antigen.

In other cases, antigen-specific immune responses may be generated against tumor cells, but the response may be too weak to eliminate the tumor. Tumors may induce immune suppression in their immediate environment, creating a type of immune-privileged site. Suppression may be mediated by suppressor lymphocytes or soluble factors, such as cytokines. Unfortunately, even though it is clear that active suppression does occur, the mechanism by which tumors mediate a suppressive environment is yet unknown.

Immune rejection and spontaneous elimination of tumors, when they do occur, appear to be due largely to the actions of antigen-specific T lymphocytes. Therefore, immunologists seeking to develop immunotherapies for cancer have focused their attentions on strategies that enhance T cell responsiveness to tumors. Some of the techniques that have been developed enhance immune responsiveness by altering the antigens expressed by tumors. Others seek to improve antigen presentation to, and costimulation of, tumor antigen-specific lymphocytes.

Immunologists have used various techniques to introduce foreign antigens into tumor cells, a process called *xenogenization* (Fig. 5-10). Harvested tumor cells may be infected with a virus or genetically manipulated to introduce a foreign gene (transfection). The infected or transfected cells, which now express foreign antigens, are reintroduced into the host, where they elicit an immune response directed against the foreign antigens. Once an immune response has been generated against the altered tumor cells, the parent tumor cells are also attacked. The exact mechanism by which this occurs is unclear, but it is probably due to cytokines that are released in the local environment of the parent cells (bystander effect).

Normal host genes may be inserted into tumor cells to enhance their immunogenicity. The most common genes that have been inserted are cytokine genes. Tumor cells often express low levels of cytokines, or they express suppressive cytokines. To overcome this tendency, genes that encode stimulatory cytokines may be introduced into the cells.

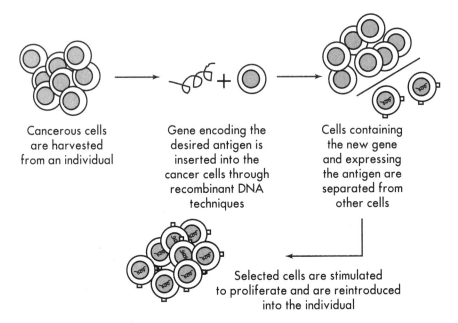

Cancerous cells are harvested from an individual

Gene encoding the desired antigen is inserted into the cancer cells through recombinant DNA techniques

Cells containing the new gene and expressing the antigen are separated from other cells

Selected cells are stimulated to proliferate and are reintroduced into the individual

Fig. 5-10 Cancerous cells that do not stimulate an immune response may be genetically manipulated to express stimulatory antigens on their cell surfaces. A gene that encodes a costimulatory molecule (e.g., B7) or a foreign protein (e.g., a viral protein) may be inserted into the DNA of the cancer cell. The altered cancer cells can then by used to induce an immune response against the entire tumor from which the cells were derived.

Interleukin-2, a key cytokine inducing lymphocytes to proliferate and become effector cells, has been shown to induce immune responses against tumors that express the cytokine. Costimulatory molecules, such as B7, are also possible targets for genetic insertion because cells expressing B7 would be more likely to activate lymphocytes that recognize antigens on their cell surfaces.

Strategies have been developed to improve presentation of cryptic (hidden) antigens. Many cancer-associated antigens are not readily accessible to the immune system, and the immune system essentially ignores them because of their location even though they are potentially immunogenic. Cryptic antigens may not be able to bind to MHC molecules and be displayed on the surface of the tumor cell. Alternatively, they may be antigens that are not readily produced by the cancer cell, being the products of "silent" genes. Tumor cells can be genetically manipulated so that their cryptic antigens are produced and presented in the proper manner on the surface of the cell, making them targets for immune attack. The drawback in manipulating cryptic antigens is that they may also be cryptic antigens in normal cells, and once an immune response is activated against them, the immune system also may attack normal cells possessing similar antigens, creating an autoimmune state.

Tumor cells also have been treated with exogenous cytokines, such as interferon-gamma, to increase their expression of MHC molecules. This has increased the immunogenicity of some tumors by enhancing their ability to present tumor antigen/MHC complexes to lymphocytes. However, increased MHC expression also can have a negative effect on immune responsiveness by inhibiting recognition of tumor cells by nonspecific immune cells, such as natural killer cells, which tend to preferentially destroy targets expressing low levels of MHC molecules.

All of the aforementioned strategies seek to enhance antigen-specific recognition of tumor cells. However, an additional strategy, called *T-cell retargeting*, bypasses the traditional requirements for antigen recognition to link nonspecific effector T cells with cancer cells. Bispecific antibodies that bind to the T-cell receptor (TCR) complex on effector T cells, as well as to a selected membrane antigen on tumor cells, are generated in vitro. These antibodies bind to the TCR in a stimulatory manner. By simultaneously binding to tumor cells and T cells, these antibodies bring tumor cells and activated lymphocytes into close physical contact. Bound, activated helper T cells secrete cytokines just as though they had been stimulated by their specific antigen, and the secreted cytokines act to inhibit or destroy the tumor cell. Bound, activated cytotoxic T cells also may affect tumor cells to which they are linked, although the mechanism by which this is accomplished in the absence of antigen-specific binding between the effector and target cells is less clear. The potential for autoimmune side effects exists for T-cell retargeting because the bispecific antibodies also may bind to normal host cells if they express similar target cell surface antigens.

Even though the advances in tumor immunology during the past decade have been substantial, they must be approached with tempered optimism. The strategies were largely developed in mice, using tumors induced by viral infection or large doses of radiation or drugs. Their applicability to spontaneous tumors in humans and domestic animals has yet to be proved. Also, the universal "cancer vaccine" is still elusive, as these strategies must be customized for each tumor and individual. It is likely that these strategies will first be tested in individuals with advanced disease, and it is possible that their cancers may be too widely disseminated (metastatic) and prolific to be responsive to immunotherapy.

However, it is possible that immunotherapy will serve as a useful adjunct to other cancer therapies, even in metastatic cases.

Related Topics

T lymphocyte antigen recognition
Costimulatory signals for lymphocytes
Tolerance

Additional Reading

Hellstrom, I. and Hellstrom, K.E. 1993. Tumor immunology: an overview. Ann. N. Y. Acad. Sci. 690:24-33.
Roth, C., Rochlitz, C., and Kourilsky, P. 1994. Immune response against tumors. Adv. Immunol. 57:281-351.

TERMS:

Immunogenic	Capable of stimulating an immune response.
Metastasis	Spread of cancer cells beyond their original tumor site.
T-cell Retargeting	Method of inducing the immune system to attack cancer cells by using antibodies to link cancer cells and lymphocytes together. The antibodies bind to the lymphocyte in a stimulatory manner so that activated lymphocytes are in close proximity to the cancer cells.
Xenogenization	The process of making a cancer cell more immunogenic by inserting a foreign gene into its nucleus. The inserted gene produces a protein that is foreign and recognizable by host lymphocytes.

Study Questions

1. How do cancer cells differ from normal cells?
2. How might cancer cells escape immune surveillance?
3. What components of the native and acquired immune systems can help to control cancer cells?
4. What are some of the methods that have been used by immunologists to increase the ability of tumor cells to be recognized by the immune system?

TOPIC 9: Immunosenescence

Principles

1. The ability of the immune system to protect against infection and cancer and to avoid autoimmune disease decreases in advanced age.
2. The immune system in different individuals undergoes age-related changes (immunosenescence) at different rates and to different degrees.
3. Some cells and functions of the immune system are more affected by age than others.

Explanation

As an individual ages, there are accompanying changes in the functions and effectiveness of many body systems. As a population, elderly individuals are more susceptible to microbial infections and do not respond as effectively as younger individuals to vaccination, observations that suggest that there are age-related changes in the immune system. Elderly individuals are also at higher risk for developing cancers, which may reflect a decrease in the efficiency of the immune system to detect and eliminate abnormal host cells.

Aging of the immune system, or *immunosenescence,* is a growing area of study for immunologists, but knowledge in this area is still limited. However, it is evident that certain aspects of immune function are more affected by age than are others, and not all commonly observed senescent changes are inevitable consequences of aging in all individuals.

The first detectable event in immunosenescence occurs around puberty, when the thymus begins to involute, becoming a small remnant of tissue by middle age. This thymic involution is probably due to hormonal changes that occur with aging, particularly the decrease in growth hormone, which has been shown to promote the maintenance of thymic tissue and to increase the production of some thymic hormones. T lymphocyte populations, which arise from the thymus, would be expected to be most heavily affected. Indeed, the absolute numbers of all T-cell subsets decrease in elderly individuals. There is also a shift in the relative proportions of various T-cell subsets, including an increase in memory cells and a decrease in virgin (naive) cells. However, the absolute number of virgin cells remains fairly constant after age 40 in humans, suggesting that perhaps the role of the thymus in producing virgin T lymphocytes may be assumed by another peripheral lymphoid tissue as an individual ages.

Lymphocytes in older individuals undergo functional changes too. Their cell membranes are often partially depolarized, which may decrease their ability to transmit certain activating signals from the external environment to the cell nucleus. They also tend to express lower levels of receptors for costimulatory signals on their cell surfaces. This may explain why T cells in aged individuals often respond poorly to antigens that normally stimulate widespread cell proliferation (polyclonal mitogens). They also express altered profiles of homing receptors and cell adhesion molecules on their cell surfaces, which may affect their ability to localize in areas of infection or inflammation. Aged lymphocytes produce less interleukin-2, a key regulatory cytokine involved in proliferation and activation of many immune cell types, and they are less responsive to its effects.

Lymphocytes in elderly individuals are more subject to gene mutations and oxidative death. Many gene mutations do not lead to cancerous conditions (unrestrained replication) but rather cause the affected cell to become nonfunctional or to die. This could contribute to the decreased immune responsiveness observed in some aged cell populations. Reactions of various cellular molecules with oxygen can lead to the generation of oxygen radicals, unstable molecules that are toxic to cells. Young lymphocytes have mechanisms to protect themselves somewhat against oxygen radicals, but they start to lose this ability with age.

Elderly individuals tend to have reduced delayed-type hypersensitivity reactions, especially to antigens to which they are exposed late in life. Consequently, they have a higher incidence of false-negative results in diagnostic tests that utilize delayed-type hypersensitivity responses, such as tuberculin tests.

With age, the immune system appears to become more focused on self antigens and less reactive to foreign antigens. Serum antibody levels remain fairly constant with aging, but the proportion of self-reactive antibodies (autoantibodies) in the blood increases. Elderly individuals have reduced antibody responses to foreign antigens, such as bacteria or viruses, although the rate and magnitude of the decline differs among antigens and host species. This reduced responsiveness can often be overcome with increased doses of antigen. Conversely, antibody responses to self antigens, which would normally be suppressed, are enhanced in older individuals. In humans, the majority of individuals older than age 65 have circulating autoantibodies. However, the presence of autoantibodies is not always associated with disease. Many individuals with circulating autoantibodies never show clinical signs of autoimmunity; autoantibodies in these individuals are not usually directed toward a specific organ. They are considered "physiological" autoantibodies and may aid in the removal of senescent or damaged host cells.

There are several possible reasons why autoantibody production is increased in elderly individuals. A particular subset of B lymphocytes, CD5+ lymphocytes, increases with age. CD5+ B lymphocytes are responsible for the production of many autoantibodies. Also, the expression of histocompatibility antigens in the thymus is reduced with age, which may decrease the stringency with which T lymphocytes are selected for their reactivity against foreign (not self) antigens. Splenic lymphocytes from aged mice tend to produce decreased amounts of T_h1-type cytokines (cytokines that enhance cell-mediated immunity) and increased amounts of T_h2-type cytokines (cytokines that enhance antibody production). This shift toward antibody-enhancing cytokines may allow low affinity self-reactive B lymphocytes that might not normally be stimulated to produce antibodies.

Immunosenescence should not be considered synonymous with immune deterioration or immune deficiency. Although some aspects of immune function are reduced in aged individuals, other parameters remain constant or are enhanced. Also, different compartments of the immune system are affected to differing degrees. For instance, few age-related changes in the mucosal immune system have been described. Additionally, not all individuals experience immunosenescence at the same rate or to the same degree. Populations of extremely old individuals, such as centenarians, tend to have a high incidence of relatively intact immune functions.

An understanding of immunosenescence has clinical applicability. Immunologists have used measurements of certain immune parameters to estimate morbidity and mortality in certain individuals. No individual immune functions can be correlated with impending mortality, but a combination of changes has been predictive in some studies. An understanding of age-related changes may also lead to the development of therapeutic strategies to retard, or even reverse, immunosenescence. Particularly critical in this area are changes resulting from dysregulation rather than dysfunction. If aged immune cells are still capable of normal responses when given the proper regulatory signals, immunologists may be able to enhance immune function through the administration of cytokines or other regulatory factors.

Additional Reading

Franceschi, C., Monti, D., Sansoni, P., and Cossarizza, A. 1995. The immunology of exceptional individuals: the lesson of centenarians. Immunol. Today. 16:12-16.

Miller, R. 1995. Cellular and biochemical changes in the aging mouse immune system. Nutr. Rev. 53:S8-S14.

Pawelec, G., Adibzadeh, M., Pohla, H., and Schaudt, K. 1995. Immunosenescence: aging of the immune system. Immunol. Today. 16:420-422.

Weksler, M. 1995. Immune senescence: deficiency or dysregulation. Nutr. Rev. 53:S3-S7.

TERMS:

Autoantibodies	Antibodies directed against self antigens.
CD5+ lymphocytes	Subset of B lymphocytes possessing the cell marker CD5. CD5+ lymphocytes are often associated with the production of autoantibodies.
Immunosenescence	Aging of the immune system.

Study Questions

1. Describe three general immunological changes that tend to occur as individuals age.
2. Why is immunosenescence distinct from immunodeficiency?
3. Describe the changes that occur in thymus structure and function from birth through old age.
4. What factors may lead to increased autoantibody production in aging individuals?

Glossary

Aberrant: Abnormal

Acute Phase Proteins: A group of proteins produced by the liver in response to infection or inflammation. They include C-reactive protein, amyloid A, fibrinogen, haptoglobin, and transferrin

Acute Phase Response: A nonspecific response to infection or inflammation characterized by the appearance of acute phase proteins in the blood

Addressins: Molecules on the surface of endothelial cells to which leukocytes adhere as they home to specific sites

Affinity: Strength of binding

Affinity Maturation: Phenomenon wherein the average affinity of a population of antibody molecules increases over time following exposure to an antigen

Agglutination: Clumping of particulate matter

Allele: One of two or more alternative forms of a gene at a specific site (locus) on a chromosome

Allelic Exclusion: Phenomenon in which only one of two genes (alleles) at a specific site on a chromosome is expressed

Alloantigens: Antigens present in some individuals within a species and not other individuals

Allograft: Transplant from one individual to a genetically different individual of the same species

Alloreactivity: An immune response against alloantigens

Allotype: A distinct antigenic type within an immunoglobulin, resulting from differences in amino acid sequences in the immunoglobulin light chains

Anaphylaxis: Severe shock-type reaction that occurs rapidly after exposure to antigen. Caused by IgE-mediated release of mediators from mast cell granules

Anergy: Diminished capacity or inability to respond to a specific antigen

Antibody-Dependent Cellular Cytotoxicity (ADCC): Leukocyte-mediated destruction of cells that have been coated with antibody

Antigen: Substance that induces an immune response and/or reacts with products of an immune response

Antigenic: Capable of inducing an immune response

Antigen Masking: The coating of certain pathogens with host proteins to avoid detection by the immune system

Antigen-Presenting Cells: Cells that are capable of processing antigens and presenting them on their surface in association with either type I or type II major histocompatibility molecules

Antigen Processing: The intracellular cleavage of protein molecules and their binding to major histocompatibility complex (MHC) molecules. Takes place within antigen-presenting cells

Antigen Sequestration: Process of isolating antigens in locations where they are not exposed to the immune system

Apoptosis: Programmed cell death, results from a signal that causes condensation of chromatin and degradation of DNA

Arthus Reaction: Local inflammatory reaction caused by the formation of antigen-antibody complexes and complement activation. A type III hypersensitivity

Atopy: An allergic hypersensitivity state caused by IgE antibodies and a hereditary predisposition

Autoantibodies: Antibodies that react with self antigens

Autoimmunity: Clinical disease caused by an immune response to self antigens

Autoreactive: Capable of reacting with self antigens

Bystander Effect: Nonspecific damage to cells or tissues caused by inflammatory products produced in a nearby specific immune response

CD Molecules: Cell surface molecules defined by the internationally recognized CD (Cluster of Differentiation) system, based on their reactivity with monoclonal antibodies

Central Tolerance: Inactivation or destruction of lymphocytes that react to a specific antigen; central tolerance occurs within primary lymphoid tissues

Chemoattractants: Small molecules that diffuse away from their site of production, forming a chemical concentration gradient that attracts certain types of cells to the area

Chemokines: Family of chemotactic cytokines

Chemotaxis: Movement of cells along a concentration of chemoattractant molecules

Class Switching: The change of antibody class (isotype) that is produced by a B lymphocyte during an immune response to a specific antigen. This occurs through rearrangement of B cell DNA coding the constant heavy chain portion of the antibody molecule

Clonal Expansion: Proliferation of one or more cells to form a larger population of identical daughter cells

Colony Stimulating Factors: Group of cytokines that regulate the formation, differentiation, and maturation of leukocytes in the bone marrow

Colostrum: First milk, present at the time of parturition. It has a high concentration of antibodies

Congenital: Present at birth

Constant Region: Region of an antibody molecule that has nearly the same amino acid sequence in all members of the same species

Constitutive: Continuously present

Costimulatory Signals: Signals received by B or T lymphocytes in addition to those transmitted through antigen binding. These signals may come from cytokines or from cell-cell contact

Cryptic Epitopes: Antigenic sites that are hidden within a molecule because of the three-dimensional structure of the intact molecule

Cytokines: Protein molecules that serve as chemical messengers between cells. They play a key role in regulating cells of the immune system

Cytotoxic T Lymphocytes: Thymus-derived lymphocytes that usually express CD8 molecules and recognize peptide antigens presented in conjunction with MHC class I molecules. These cells can directly kill antigen-presenting cells and can secrete cytokines

Dendritic Cells: Specialized mononuclear phagocytic cells with long cytoplasmic processes. Found in skin (Langerhans cells) and lymph nodes, they function as antigen trapping and presenting cells

Double Negative Lymphocytes: T lymphocytes that have neither CD4 nor CD8 molecules on their surface

Double Positive Lymphocytes: T lymphocytes that have both CD4 and CD8 molecules on their surface

Effector Cells: Cells of the immune system that are able to bring about an effect, such as cytotoxic T lymphocytes, activated macrophages, and natural killer cells

Endogenous Pathway of Antigen Processing: Processing of proteins located within the cell cytoplasm into small peptides, binding those peptides to class I MHC molecules, and presenting the MHC-peptide complexes on the cell surface

Epitope: Area on an antigen molecule that directly binds to an antibody molecule or T-lymphocyte receptor. Synonymous with antigenic determinant

Exogenous Pathway of Antigen Processing: Processing of endocytosed proteins into small peptides, binding those peptides to class II MHC molecules, and presenting the MHC-peptide complexes on the cell surface

Extravasation: Process whereby a leukocyte migrates through the vascular wall

Fab Fragment: Antigen binding portion of an antibody molecule that is produced when antibodies are digested with papain

Fas: A cell membrane receptor for the tumor necrosis factor family of cytokines. Cross-linking of Fas receptors leads to cell death (apoptosis)

Fc Fragment: The "crystallizable" fragment of an immunoglobulin after papain digestion. This portion of the Ig molecule cannot bind antigen, but it is responsible for most of the biological activity of immunoglobulin molecules

Fibrin: Insoluble protein that forms the basis of a blood clot

Fibroblasts: Cells that form the connective tissues of the body

Gamma/Delta T Lymphocyte: T lymphocytes possessing the gamma/delta form of T-cell receptor rather than the conventional alpha/beta form. They are often abundant in the lamina propria of the gut and may play a role in mucosal immunity

Germinal Center: Areas in lymphoid tissue where B lymphocytes undergo mitosis after antigenic stimulation

Glomerulonephritis: Inflammation of the glomeruli of the kidney

Graft vs. Host Disease: A clinical condition in which lymphocytes from transplanted tissues attack the tissues of an immunocompromised recipient

Granzymes: A family of proteases found in the granules of cytotoxic T lymphocytes and natural killer cells

Graves Disease: Hyperplasia of the thyroid, leading to hyperthyroidism. Some cases are due to the formation of autoantibodies against the receptor for thyroid-stimulating hormone (TSH); the antibodies mimic the action of TSH

Heat Shock Proteins: Group of highly conserved cellular proteins that are produced by cells in response to heat and other stressors. They play a role in protein assembly and protein transport within a cell

Helper T Lymphocytes: Thymus-derived lymphocytes that usually have CD4 molecules on their surface and recognize antigen presented on major histocompatibility complex class II molecules. They secrete cytokines and help other immune cells respond to antigen

Hematopoietic Organs: Organs in which blood cells are produced

Hemolysis: Lysis or destruction of red blood cells

Hepatic: A term referring to the liver

High Endothelial Venules: Postcapillary venules with cuboidal epithelial cells, found in the paracortex of lymph nodes. Lymphocytes leave the blood and enter the lymph node through these vessels

Homodimer: A molecule composed of two identical subunits

HPA Axis: Hypothalamic-pituitary-adrenal axis. The interactions that occur between the hypothalamus in the brain, the pituitary gland at the base of the brain, and the adrenal gland near the kidney play an important role in the response to stress

Hypersensitivity Disease: Those diseases in which an excessive or inappropriate immune response is responsible for clinical signs

Hypervariable Regions: Small regions within immunoglobulin and T-cell receptor molecules in which the greatest variations in amino acid sequence occur. These are the regions that contact antigen molecules and define antigen specificity

Hyposensitization: A technique to reduce the response to certain antigens involved in hypersensitivity disease. It usually refers to the administration of an allergen via an atypical route in an attempt to reduce IgE production

ICAMs: Intercellular adhesion molecules. ICAMs facilitate and mediate certain cell-cell interactions

Idiotype: Classification type for antibody molecules, based on the portions of an antibody molecule that determine antigenic specificity

Immunocompetence: The ability of an individual to produce an immune response

Immunogenic: Capable of eliciting an immune response in an individual

Immunoglobulin Domains: Regions in immunoglobulin light and heavy chains, consisting of approximately 100 amino acids and an intrachain disulfide bond. Amino acid sequences among domains are somewhat conserved, so domains are also referred to as homology regions

Immunological Memory: Capacity of the immune system to react more quickly and aggressively against antigens to which it has previously been exposed

Immunomodulation: Manipulation of the immune system, usually enhancement of immune responses

Immunopathology: Study of tissue damage caused by inappropriate immune responses

Immunosenescence: Aging of the immune system

In Utero: Within the uterus

Integrins: Family of molecules that mediate firm binding of leukocytes to blood vessel walls

Interferons: Family of cytokines known for its antiviral properties and its ability to activate many types of immune cells

Interleukin: Family of cytokines, originally defined as those cytokines used for cellular communication between leukocytes but now known also to affect nonleukocyte cells

Intradermal: Within the skin

Intraepithelial Lymphocytes: Lymphocytes scattered among the epithelial cells on the surface of various body surfaces

Invariant Complex: Portion of a lymphocyte antigen receptor that is highly conserved among animal species; includes the CD3 molecule and associated protein chains

Involution: Degeneration, shrinkage

Isotype: Antibody class, such as IgG, IgM, IgA, IgD, or IgE

Jaundice: Yellowish discoloration of the skin and mucous membranes caused by accumulation of bile in the tissues

Junctional Diversity: Variability among antigen receptors that is introduced through the laxity in the site where gene segments may join together

Kupffer Cells: Nonmigratory macrophages located within the vasculature of the liver

LAK Cells: Lymphokine-activated killer cells; natural killer lymphocytes that have been stimulated by cytokines so that they have an enhanced ability to kill foreign or neoplastic cells

Lamina Propria: Layer of connective tissue within the intestine and other mucosal surfaces that lies directly beneath the surface layer of epithelial cells

Latent: Dormant, inactive; lying hidden

Leukocyte Adhesion Deficiency (LAD): Primary immunodeficiency in which leukocytes cannot effectively reach sites of inflammation because they lack the adhesive molecules to exit the bloodstream. Individuals with LAD suffer from recurrent bacterial infections

Leukocyte Trafficking: Controlled process by which leukocytes adhere to the walls of blood vessels and exit the bloodstream

Ligand: Complementary molecule to which a receptor molecule binds

Lymph: A fluid, rich in lymphocytes, derived from tissue fluids. Lymph circulates in lymphatic vessels before being released into the bloodstream

Lymphocyte Homing: Phenomenon wherein lymphocytes originating from a particular tissue tend to return to that tissue after circulating in the blood and lymph

Lymphokine: Cytokine, specifically those cytokines secreted by lymphocytes

Major Histocompatibility Complex (class I and II): A gene region that encodes proteins that mediate graft rejection and aid in presentation of antigens to lymphocytes

Malaise: General feeling of ill-being, characterized by fatigue, lethargy, and discomfort

Metastatic: Disseminated from an original focus, such as cancer cells that spread from a primary tumor

Mitogens: Substances that stimulate cells to undergo mitosis (divide)

Motility: Ability to move

Mucosal: Covered by a mucous membrane

Mucosal-Associated Lymphoid Tissue (MALT): Scattered foci of lymphoid tissue that are located beneath mucosal surfaces, such as in the intestine, respiratory tract, and reproductive tract

Naive: Unexposed; has not encountered a given antigen

Necrosis: Cell death

Negative Thymic Selection: Process within the thymus wherein lymphocytes that react against self antigens are eliminated

Neonatal Isoerythrolysis: Condition in which the immune system of a neonate attacks the individual's own red blood cells because maternally derived antibodies have bound to paternal antigens on the cells

Neurotransmitter: Chemical that transmits signals between nerve cells

Neutropenia: Deficiency of neutrophils in the bloodstream; may be relative or absolute

Noncovalent Bond: Bond between two molecules that does not involve sharing of electrons

Omentum: Tissue that lies between abdominal organs and the body wall; the omentum can mold around organs and tissues to localize areas of inflammation or infection

Opsonization: Process of coating a cell or particle with antibodies and/or complement so that the particle can be more efficiently internalized by phagocytic cells

Oral Tolerance: Immunological phenomenon wherein foreign antigens introduced orally are tolerated by the immune system. Introduction of the same antigens through parenteral routes would stimulate an immune response

Oxidation: Chemical reaction that results in the loss of an electron

Oxygen Radicals: Unstable forms of oxygen (usually through the gain or loss of electrons) that are generated within phagocytic cells; exposure to oxygen radicals is lethal to many cells and infectious agents

Paratope: Portion of an antibody molecule that binds with an epitope on an antigen

Parenchymal Cells: Organ-specific cells that make up the substance of that organ

Pathogenic: Capable of causing disease

Pathological: Diseased

Perforin: Protein that mediates cytotoxicity by lymphocytes; perforin forms pores within cellular membranes

Perinatal: Around the time of birth

Peripheral Tolerance: Immunological nonresponsiveness to a given antigen that is established outside of primary lymphoid tissues (i.e., thymus, bone marrow)

Peyer's Patches: Organized lymphoid tissue located along the length of the intestine

Phagocytosis: Process of internalizing particulate matter by cells

Phenotype: Collective term for outward characteristics associated with the possession and expression of a gene

Pituitary: Endocrine gland located at the base of the brain that regulates many nervous and hormonal processes; also called the "master gland" of the brain

Placenta: Tissue that surrounds and supports development of a fetus within the uterus

Plasma Cells: B lymphocytes that have transformed into cells optimized for antibody secretion

Polyclonal Mitogens: Substances that stimulate lymphocytes to divide in a non–antigen-specific manner

Polymorphic: Having many forms

Positive Thymic Selection: Process within the thymus wherein lymphocytes that recognize foreign antigens in combination with self major histocompatibility molecules are rescued from cell death and/or allowed to mature

Precipitation: Association of molecules into aggregates large enough to fall out of solution

Precursor: Forebearer; precursor cells are immature cells that undergo additional development before becoming functional

Primary Immunodeficiency: Lack of immune function or immune dysfunction because of an inherent defect in the immune system

Primary Lymphoid Tissue: Tissue where lymphocytes mature and undergo selection; includes the thymus, bone marrow, bursa of Fabricius (birds), and ileocecal lymph nodes (ruminants)

Prophylactic: Preventive

Proteinase: Also called protease; enzyme that degrades proteins

Pruritis: Itching sensation

Psychoneuroimmunology: Study of the combined effects and interactions among the nervous system, immune system, and behavior

Secondary Immunodeficiency: Lack of immune function or immune dysfunction because of an acquired defect (viral infection, injury, degeneration) in the immune system

Secondary Lymphoid Tissue: Lymphoid tissue, scattered throughout the body, where antigens and lymphocytes interact; includes most lymph nodes and disseminated lymphoid tissue (e.g. MALT)

Second Set Reaction: Accelerated rejection of transplanted foreign tissue that occurs when an individual has been previously sensitized to antigens of the tranplanted tissue

Selectins: Molecules that facilitate adhesion of leukocytes to vascular walls; selectins mediate initial binding between leukocytes and endothelium

Sequestration: Process of walling off or isolating something from its surroundings

Serum Sickness: Generalized form of type III hypersensitivity

Shear Force: Tearing force that is generated when two substances move in a parallel manner against each other

Silencer Gene: Gene that prevents the expression of another associated gene

Somatic Mutation: Alteration of gene sequence in mature cells, usually by incorporation of an incorrect nucleic acid during DNA replication during mitosis

Stress Proteins: Proteins produced by cells during times of physiological stress; stress proteins are primitive and highly conserved in structure across evolutionarily distinct cell types

Substrate: Substance upon which enzymes act

Subunit Vaccine: Immunizing product that is composed of selected antigens from an infectious agent rather than the intact agent

Superantigens: Select group of antigens that bind to lymphocytes in an atypical manner and that may stimulate large populations of lymphocytes to proliferate and secrete cytokines

Sympathetic Nerves: Subgroup of peripheral nerves involved in "fight or flight" responses

Synapse: Junction between two nerve cells

Systemic Lupus Erythematosus (SLE): Generalized autoimmune disease characterized by type III hypersensitivity

T-Cell Retargeting: Method of inducing the immune system to attack cancer cells by using antibodies to link cancer cells and lymphocytes together

TCR: T-cell receptor; antigen receptor found on the surface of T lymphocytes

Tethering: A component of the leukocyte trafficking process wherein the leukocyte loosely attaches to a blood vessel wall

T_h0 Lymphocytes: Subset of helper T lymphocytes that do not fit into the category of Th1 or Th2 lymphocytes

T_h1 Lymphocytes: Subset of helper T lymphocytes that secrete cytokines that promote cell-mediated immune processes

T_h2 Lymphocytes: Subset of helper T lymphocytes that secrete cytokines that promote antibody production

Thrombi: Blood clots within a blood vessel

Thymic Selection: Process of sorting lymphocytes that recognize foreign antigens from those that are reactive against self antigens; characterized by positive and negative selection processes

Thymotrophic: Stimulatory or enhancing to the thymus

Tissue Typing: Process of comparing major histocompatibility molecules between donor and recipient tissues to determine suitability for transplantation

Titer: In immunology, a measurement of antibody concentration

Tolerance: Immune nonresponsiveness; may be absolute or relative, temporary or permanent

Toxic Shock Syndrome: Generalized physiological shock caused by massive release of cytokines into the circulation; associated with superantigens such as *Staphylococcus* toxins

Transfection: Uptake of DNA into a cell

Transforming Growth Factors: Family of cytokines that mediates healing and repair processes; originally characterized by their ability to transform the phenotype of cultured cells

Transgenic Animals: Animals that, through recombinant DNA technology, possess selected genes derived from another animal species

Transplacental: Across the placental membrane

Transudate: Intercellular fluid that has passed through a cell membrane and is low in protein

Triggering: Component of leukocyte trafficking process wherein loosely adherent leukocytes are stimulated to bind firmly to the wall of blood vessels

Tumor Necrosis Factor: Proinflammatory cytokine that is secreted early during inflammatory and infectious processes; originally characterized by its ability to mediate destruction of certain tumor cells

Tumor Surveillance: A function of the immune system wherein cells expressing abnormal antigens are destroyed and removed from the body

Type (or class) I Hypersensitivity: Also called immediate hypersensitivity; an exaggerated immune response caused by IgE that occurs within minutes of exposure to certain antigens, characterized by release of histamine and other vasoactive substances from mast cells and basophils

Type (or class) II Hypersensitivity: An exaggerated immune response caused by antibodies that bind to nonsoluble antigen (usually cell-bound). Antigen-antibody complexes activate complement, leading to cell lysis by the membrane attack complex of complement

Type (or class) III Hypersensitivity: Also called immune complex hypersensitivity; an exaggerated immune response caused by antibodies that bind to soluble antigen. The antigen-antibody complexes are deposited in small vessels, attracting neutrophils and other inflammatory factors that mediate tissue damage

Type (or class) IV Hypersensitivity: Also called delayed type hypersensitivity; an exaggerated immune response that occurs 24 to 72 hours after exposure to certain antigens, characterized by an accumulation of mononuclear inflammatory cells (macrophages, lymphocytes) at the inflammatory site

Variable Regions: Portions of antibody molecules where the sequence of amino acids differs moderately from other antibody molecules from the same species of animal; contrasts with constant regions, which have less variability, and hypervariable regions, which are more variable

Vasculitis: Inflammation of blood vessels

VCAMs: Family of molecules located on vascular endothelial cells that mediate binding of leukocytes

Wheals: Localized, smooth swelling of the skin, which may be reddened or pale and usually itches; most often the result of a type I hypersensitivity

Xenogenization: Process whereby a tissue is altered so that it expresses antigens foreign to the host

Xenograft: Transplanted tissue derived from a different animal species than the recipient individual

Yolk Sac: Primitive embryonic structure from which immune cell precursors may arise

Index

NORTHERN MICHIGAN UNIVERSITY

3 1854 005 843 589